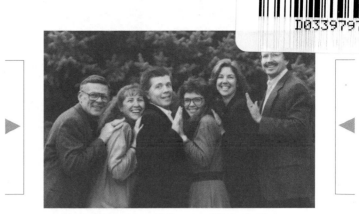

Our "Compacted" Compact Clinicals Team

Dear Valued Customer,

WELCOME to Compact Clinicals. We are committed to bringing mental health professionals up-to-date diagnostic and treatment information in a compact, timesaving, and easy-to-read format. Our line of books provides current, thorough reviews of assessment and treatment strategies for mental disorders.

We've "compacted" complete information for diagnosing each disorder and comparing how different theoretical orientations approach treatment. Our books use nonacademic language, real-world examples, and well-defined terminology.

Enjoy this and other timesaving books from Compact Clinicals.

Sincerely,

Melanie A. Dean

Melanie Dean, Ph.D.
President

Compact Clinicals Line of Books

Compact Clinicals currently offers these condensed reviews for professionals:

For Clinicians

Attention Deficit Hyperactivity Disorder
The latest assessment and treatment strategies

C. Keith Conners, Ph.D.

Bipolar Disorder
The latest assessment and treatment strategies

Trisha Suppes M.D., Ph.D., and Ellen B. Dennehy, Ph.D.

Borderline Personality Disorder
The latest assessment and treatment strategies

Melanie Dean, Ph.D.

Conduct Disorders
The latest assessment and treatment strategies

J. Mark Eddy, Ph.D.

Depression in Adults
The latest assessment and treatment strategies

Anton Tolman, Ph.D.

Obsessive Compulsive Disorder
The latest assessment and treatment strategies

Gail Steketee, Ph.D., and Teresa Pigot, M.D.

Post-Traumatic and Acute Stress Disorders
The latest assessment and treatment strategies

Matthew Friedman, M.D., Ph.D.

For Physicians

Bipolar Disorder: Treatment and Management
Trisha Suppes, M.D., Ph.D., and Paul E. Keck, Jr., M.D.

Post-Traumatic and Acute Stress Disorders

The latest assessment and treatment strategies

Fourth Edition

Matthew Friedman, M.D., Ph.D.

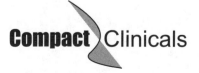

This book is intended for use by properly trained and licensed mental health professionals, who already possess a solid education in psychological theory, research, and treatment. This book is in no way intended to replace or supplement such training and education, nor is it to be used as the sole basis for any decision regarding treatment. It is merely intended to be used by such trained and educated professionals as a review and resource guide when considering how to best treat a person with post-traumatic stress disorder or an acute stress disorder.

Post-Traumatic and Acute Stress Disorders

The latest assessment and treatment strategies

Fourth Edition

by

Matthew Friedman, M.D., Ph.D.

Compact Clinicals

Published by: Compact Clinicals
7205 NW Waukomis Dr., Suite A
Kansas City, MO 64151
816-587-0044

©2006 Dean Psych Press Corp. d/b/a Compact Clinicals
Prior Releases: ©2000, 2001, 2003 Dean Psych Press Corp. d/b/a Compact Clinicals

Medical Editing: Kathi L. Whitman, In Credible English, Inc.® Kansas City, Missouri
Book Design: Coleridge Design, Kansas City, Missouri

Library of Congress Cataloging in Publication data:

Friedman, Matthew
Post-traumatic and acute stress disorders : the latest assessment and treatment strategies / by Matthew Friedman.
        p.   ; cm.
    Includes bibliographical references and index.
    ISBN 1-887537-22-8
    1. Post-traumatic stress disorder. 2. Post-traumatic stress disorder – Treatment.
I. Title.
    RC552.P67F749 2006
    616.85'2106–dc22
            2005009024

10 9 8 7 6 5 4 3 2 1

From the Author

Despite the new title, this book is really an updated version of *Post-Traumatic Stress Disorder: The Latest Assessment and Treatment Strategies,* first published by Compact Clinicals in 2000 and revised twice, since then.

The change in title and organization has been prompted primarily by what has happened in the field as a result of the terrorist attacks of September 11, 2001. Since that time, a great deal of attention has been devoted to understanding both adaptive and pathological acute responses to traumatic events. Such efforts have generated important conceptual and clinical advances from both a public health and more traditional clinical perspective.

Therefore, the last chapter is devoted entirely to acute post-traumatic reactions, while the first five chapters focus entirely on PTSD. We have chosen this sequence for two, key reasons:

1. The PTSD material is the fundamental context through which all the acute material is best understood.

2. The scientific and clinical bases for PTSD are well established, while the acute field is in a much more preliminary phase of development.

Thank you for opening this book. I hope that it will hold your attention, adequately address your major questions, and enhance your ability to recognize, diagnose, and treat PTSD and acute post-traumatic reactions.

Sincerely,

Matthew J. Friedman M.D., Ph.D.

From the Publisher

As a mental health professional, often the information you need can only be obtained after countless hours of reading or library research. If your schedule precludes this time commitment, Compact Clinicals is the answer.

Our books are practitioner oriented with easy-to-read treatment descriptions and examples. Compact Clinicals books are written in a nonacademic style. Our books are formatted to make the first reading, as well as ongoing reference, quick and easy. You will find:

▶ *Anecdotes* — Each chapter contains a fictionalized account that personalizes the disorder entitled, "From the Patient's Perspective."

▶ *Sidebars* — Narrow columns on the outside of each page highlight important information, preview upcoming sections or concepts, and define terms used in the text.

▶ *Definitions* — Terms are defined in the sidebars where they originally appear in the text and in an alphabetical glossary on pages 93 through 96.

▶ *References* — Numbered references appear in the text following information from that source. Full references appear on pages 97 through 110.

▶ *Case Examples* — Our examples illustrate typical client presentations that help clarify diagnosis and different treatment approaches [see pages 12–14 for detailed examples that help clarify each of the DSM-IV(TR) criteria for PTSD]. Identifying information in the examples (e.g., the individual's real name, profession, age, and/or location) has been changed to protect the confidentiality of those clients discussed in case examples.

▶ *Key Concepts* — At the end of each chapter, we include a review list of key concepts from that chapter. Use these lists for ongoing quick reference as well as for reviewing what you learned from reading the chapter.v

Contents

Chapter Four: Psychological Treatments for PTSD   33

Chapter Five: Pharmacological Treatments for PTSD   51

Chapter One:
Overview of Post-Traumatic Stress Disorder (PTSD)

This chapter answers the following:

- ▶ **What is Trauma?** — This section defines trauma, the necessary precursor to PTSD.
- ▶ **What is the History and Prevalence of PTSD?** — This section reviews how PTSD has been viewed since ancient times and presents information on how common PTSD is worldwide.
- ▶ **What are the Main Characteristics of PTSD?** — This section provides an overview of the three types of symptoms PTSD sufferers experience: reexperiencing, avoidant/numbing, and hyperarousal.
- ▶ **Can PTSD be Prevented?** — This section offers recommendations for promoting resilience among those at risk for PTSD.
- ▶ **How Severe and Chronic is PTSD?** — This section identifies three general categories of PTSD sufferers: those with lifetime PTSD, those in remission but experiencing occasional relapses, and those with delayed onset.

DURING the course of a lifetime, approximately half of all Americans will be exposed to at least one traumatic event, such as assault, military combat, an industrial or vehicular accident, rape, domestic violence, or a natural disaster (e.g., earthquake). As might be expected, exposure to extreme stress is much higher for people living in nations subjected to war, state terrorism, or forced migration, such as Algeria, Cambodia, Palestine, or Iraq. Most people can absorb the psychological impact of such an experience and resume their normal lives; however, a sizeable number cannot.

Approximately eight percent of Americans and 20 to 30 percent elsewhere (in areas of conflict) will suffer from PTSD.[1, 2]

Post-Traumatic Stress Disorder (PTSD) describes the condition a person experiences when trauma-related symptoms or impairments in everyday functioning last for at least a month and sometimes for life. PTSD has been recognized by many other names since antiquity and by modern psychiatry since the late 1800s. Although the specific symptoms included in the original PTSD diagnostic criteria have been partially modified, the fundamental PTSD construct has clearly withstood the test of time. As a result, clinicians have had 25 years in which to utilize PTSD as a diagnostic tool and to develop effective treatments.

PTSD was first defined as a distinct psychiatric diagnosis in 1980 when the American Psychiatric Association published its revised diagnostic manual, the Diagnostic and Statistical Manual of Mental Disorders-Third Edition (DSM-III).[3]

Although PTSD can only be diagnosed one month after an individual has been exposed to trauma, many people experience great distress during the immediate aftermath of a traumatic event, including having nightmares and avoiding people and places that may remind them of the trauma. Such acute, post-traumatic reactions will be considered subsequently in chapter six.

1

What is Trauma?

For a list of the specific diagnostic criteria for PTSD, see page 10.

When "trauma" was first introduced as a construct in the DSM-III diagnostic criteria for PTSD, it was defined as a catastrophic stressor that "would evoke significant symptoms of distress in most people."[3] Trauma was thought to be a rare and overwhelming event — "generally outside the range of usual human experience" — that differed qualitatively from "common experiences, such as: bereavement, chronic illness, business losses, or marital conflict." Traumatic events cited in DSM-III included: rape, assault, torture, incarceration in a death camp, military combat, natural disasters, industrial/vehicular accidents, or exposure to war/civil/domestic violence.

Initially, it was thought that trauma could be defined exclusively in terms of catastrophic events that happened to an individual who was in the wrong place at the wrong time. As initially conceptualized, anyone who had been exposed to war, rape, torture, or natural disaster, had been "traumatized."[3] This was changed in the 1994 DSM-IV [and retained in the 2000 DSM-IV (TR)] because it had become apparent that most people exposed to catastrophic events did not develop PTSD.[4, 5]

Although exposure to catastrophic stress is a necessary condition, it is not sufficient by itself to "traumatize" an individual. What also matters is the emotional response of the person exposed to such an event. If the rape or accident produced an intense emotional response [characterized in DSM-IV (TR) as "fear, helplessness, or horror"], the event is "traumatic." If an intense emotional response is not experienced, then the event is not considered a "traumatic event"; therefore, by DSM definition, the event cannot cause PTSD.

From the Patient's Perspective

That lawyer called again. He thinks I've got a great case against the trucking company and could win a huge settlement. It's tempting. I certainly need the money. But every time I even think about the accident (like now), I go to pieces. And — if I start to talk about it, I get terrified. Then the nightmares. No sleep. That horrible jumpy feeling. And I turn into a nervous wreck. It isn't worth it, even if I could win a million bucks! I'll just have to call him back tomorrow and tell him I'm not interested. He'll have to find someone else to sue.

Today, our understanding about trauma has changed significantly from that first described in the DSM-III, essentially focusing on the realizations that:

▶ **Catastrophic events are not rare.** Research has shown that over half of all American men (60.7 percent) and women (51.2 percent) are likely to be exposed to at least one catastrophic event during their lives.[1] Exposure is much higher in countries torn by war, civil strife, genocide, state-sponsored terrorism, or other forms of violence. For example, exposure to trauma was reportedly as high as 92 percent in Algeria, where deadly conflict and violence have persisted for years.[2]

▶ **Trauma is not just an external event.** The concept of trauma has changed from being considered a rare external event (DSM-III) to an individual's psychological response to a not-uncommon, overwhelming event (DSM-IV). Only people who respond to catastrophic events with fear, helplessness, or horror have been "traumatized" as defined in DSM-IV (TR).

> From a global perspective, exposure to catastrophic stress is a common fact of life.

> Fifty-four percent of American women who were raped did **not** develop PTSD; 91 percent of American women involved in an accident did **not** develop PTSD.[1]

What is the History and Prevalence of PTSD?

Historically, poets and writers have recognized that exposure to trauma may produce enduring psychological consequences. Various literary works — Homer's *Iliad*, Shakespeare's *Henry IV*, Dickens' *Tale of Two Cities* — present characters' psychological transformations and symptoms related to trauma. Even Harry Potter was perhaps traumatized when, as an infant, he witnessed his parents' murder by the evil wizard, Lord Voldemort.[6]

Historical Overview

In the late 19th century, clinical attention began to focus on the psychological impact of military combat among veterans of the U.S. Civil War and the Franco-Prussian War. Clinical formulations on both sides of the Atlantic focused either on cardiovascular (e.g., soldier's heart, Da Costa's syndrome, neurocirculatory asthenia) or psychiatric (e.g., nostalgia, shell shock, combat fatigue, war neurosis) symptoms.[7, 8] Similar clinical presentations among 19th century civilian survivors of train accidents were called "Railway Spine."[9] Throughout this period, clinicians asked to provide treatment for survivors of military or civilian trauma were struck by the physiological and psychological symptoms exhibited. Indeed, Abram Kardiner, an American psychiatrist who worked extensively with World War I veterans suffering from "War Neurosis," was so impressed by their excessive startle reaction that he called it a *"physioneurosis."*[10]

> Chapter five reviews some of the major biological abnormalities that are central to this disorder.

> **physioneurosis** — a label for the clinically significant physiological as well as psychological changes believed to be part of the "war neurosis" syndrome

Prevalence

With the growing recognition that catastrophic stress and traumatic events are much more common than originally suspected, it is clear that PTSD is a significant public health problem. Although over half of all American adults will have been exposed to a catastrophic stress (60 percent men and 51 percent women), only eight percent (five percent men and 10 percent women) will have developed PTSD at some point in their lives.[1] This means that millions of Americans will suffer from this disorder, and PTSD is a major public health problem in the U.S. and elsewhere. If untreated, many of these individuals will never recover. Research with veterans of World War II and survivors of the Nazi Holocaust has shown, for example, that PTSD can persist for over 50 years or for a lifetime.[11]

Worldwide, the psychological and physical consequences of traumatic exposure constitute a major public health challenge.[12, 13] The long-term impacts of the earthquake and tsunami disasters in Indonesia are overwhelming, both for survivors and for aid workers. Many more individuals will be exposed to trauma from nations in conflict, such as: Iraq, Afghanistan, and Rwanda as well as Algeria, Palestine, and Bosnia.[14] We must also consider the millions of children and adults exposed to sexual, physical, domestic, criminal, urban, terrorist, and genocidal violence. From this perspective, it is very important to search for effective psychological preventions and to consider providing them to children and adults as part of a global public health strategy.

What are the Main Characteristics of PTSD?

Figure 1.1, on the facing page, provides an overview of these symptom clusters.

PTSD consists of three symptom "clusters" — reexperiencing, avoidant/numbing, and hyperarousal — as well as criteria for how persistent and severe those symptoms might be that occur following a traumatic event. Chapter two provides complete DSM-IV (TR) criteria for PTSD.

Reexperiencing Symptoms

Reexperiencing can elicit symptoms of psychological distress (e.g., terror) or abnormal physiological reactions (e.g., racing pulse, rapid breathing, or sweating).

Unique to PTSD, these symptoms reflect the persistence of thoughts, feelings, and behaviors specifically related to the traumatic event. Such recollections are intrusive because they are not only unwanted but are also powerful enough to negate consideration of anything else. Daytime recollections and traumatic nightmares often evoke panic, terror, dread, grief, or despair.

Figure 1.1   PTSD Symptom Clusters

Cluster	Specific Symptoms
Reexperiencing	• Intrusive recollections • Traumatic nightmares • PTSD flashbacks • Trauma-related, stimulus-evoked psychological distress • Trauma-related, stimulus-evoked physiological reactions
Avoidant/ Numbing	• Avoiding trauma-related thoughts and feelings • Avoiding trauma-related activities, places, and people • Amnesia for trauma-related memories • Diminished interest • Feeling detached or estranged • Restricted range of affect • Sense of foreshortened future
Hyperarousal	• Insomnia • Irritability • Difficulty concentrating • Hypervigilance • Exaggerated startle reaction

Sometimes people with PTSD are exposed to reminders of the trauma (trauma-related stimuli) and are suddenly thrust into a psychological state — the PTSD flashback — in which they relive the traumatic experience, losing all connection with the present. This is referred to as an acute dissociative or brief psychotic state, in which they actually behave as if they must fight for their lives, as was the case during exposure to the initial trauma.

For example, a woman was raped at dusk by an assailant who sprang out of the shadows opening onto an urban thoroughfare. He dragged her into the recesses of a dark alley before beginning his sexual assault. It is now many months later. She is walking home from work. The setting sun produces shadows over every nook and cranny adjacent to the sidewalk. As she glances into a heavily shadowed alley, she actually "sees" an assailant poised and ready to grab her. In fact, no one is there. The similarity between the rape scene several months ago and those produced today by an urban sunset have produced a hallucination that is, in effect, a PTSD flashback. As a result, she believes that she is, again, about to be raped and runs down the street, screaming in terror.

Chapter two *reviews specific diagnostic criteria for PTSD as well as assessment strategies and instruments.* **Chapter three** *considers global treatment issues, while* **chapters four and five** *review psychological and pharmacological treatments (respectively) for PTSD.* **Chapter six** *considers acute post-traumatic reactions, including diagnostic criteria, assessment strategies, and treatment for acute stress disorder (ASD).*

Avoidant/Numbing Symptoms

These symptoms can be understood as behavioral, cognitive, or emotional strategies used to ward off the terror and distress caused by reexperiencing symptoms.

Avoidant symptoms include:

psychogenic amnesia — the inability to remember emotionally charged events for psychological rather than neurological reasons

> ► Efforts to avoid thoughts, feelings, activities, places, and people related to the original traumatic event

> ► *Psychogenic amnesia* for trauma-related memories (e.g., a 10-year-old refugee who witnessed the massacre of his father and brothers and the rape of his mother by paramilitary militia members only remembers that the troops came to the house, that he ran, hid, and eventually escaped; cannot remember what happened in between)

Numbing symptoms are psychological mechanisms through which PTSD sufferers anesthetize themselves against the intolerable panic, terror, and pain evoked by reexperiencing symptoms. These include *psychic numbing*, in which the person suppresses all feelings in order to block out the intolerable ones. This can come at a very high price (e.g., numbing intolerable, trauma-related feelings requires also anesthetizing loving feelings necessary to sustain an intimate relationship).

psychic numbing — the inability to feel any emotions, either positive (love and pleasure) or negative (fear or guilt), also described as an "emotional anesthesia"

Hyperarousal Symptoms

These symptoms are the most apparent manifestations of the excessive physiologic arousal that is part of the PTSD syndrome and include insomnia, irritability, *startle reactions,* and *hypervigilance.* Hyperarousal symptoms make up a *hyper-reactive psychophysiological state* that makes it very difficult for people with PTSD to concentrate or perform other cognitive tasks. For example, a PTSD youth might not be able to do schoolwork or focus on intellectual tasks.

startle reactions — "jumpy" behavior manifested as a tendency to exhibit an exaggerated startle response to unexpected noises or movements by others

hypervigilance — preoccupied by watchful or protective behavior motivated by excessive fears for personal safety

hyper-reactive psychophysiological state — a state in which emotions are heightened and aroused and even minor events may produce a state in which the heart pounds rapidly, muscles are tense, and there is great, overall agitation

This cluster of PTSD symptoms most closely resembles symptoms seen in *panic disorder* and *generalized anxiety disorder* and is one reason why PTSD has been classified in DSM-IV (TR) as an anxiety disorder. For information on distinguishing panic disorder and generalized anxiety disorder from PTSD, see pages 18–19.

continued

Can PTSD be Prevented?

Given the impossibility of successfully preventing traumatic events, the next best approach would be to promote **resilience** — a type of psychological "vaccine" — at the societal, community, family, and individual levels. Epidemiologic research consistently indicates that people differ in their vulnerability to (or resilience against) post-traumatic distress, supporting public mental health strategies that identify and promote resilience among those at

greatest risk for such severe, chronic, and debilitating post-traumatic reactions. Promoting resilience could mean:

▶ **At the societal level**, developing laws, policies, and
practices that ensure optimal preparation for and public
responses to terrorist attacks

▶ **At the community level**, perhaps the most effective
psychological "vaccine" for most children and adults
would be proactive psychoeducation provided in school,
workplace, and community settings

▶ **At the family level**, fostering cohesion and mutual support to help the family unit buffer the impact of traumatic
stress on its individual members

▶ **At the individual level**, enhancing the capacity of individuals to cope with traumatic stress through adaptive
strategies, such as: protective behaviors, control of physiological responses, or actively seeking social support [15]

How Severe and Chronic is PTSD?

PTSD is no different than other medical or psychiatric disorders
in that its severity may vary from mild to severe. As with dia-
betes, heart disease, and depression, some people with PTSD
can lead full and rewarding lives despite the disorder. Although
there are no current statistics, it appears that a significant minority of patients may develop a persistent, incapacitating mental
illness marked by severe and intolerable symptoms; marital,
social, and vocational disability; and extensive use of psychiatric
and community services. Such people can typically be found
on the fringes of society, in homeless shelters, or enrolled in
public-sector programs designed for people with persistent
mental illnesses, such as *schizophrenia,* from which they are
superficially indistinguishable as having PTSD. [16]

The long-term course for most people with chronic PTSD is marked
by remissions and relapses. Some people make a full recovery,
others partial improvement, and others never improve.

There are three general classes of PTSD sufferers:

1. **Lifetime PTSD** — Current surveys indicate that 40
percent of patients with *lifetime PTSD* are unlikely to
recover whether or not they have ever received treatment. [1] Some may show some improvement in functional
capacity or symptom severity, but their PTSD remains
chronic, severe, and permanent. It should be understood,
however, that effective treatments were not generally
available when this survey was conducted.

2. **PTSD in Remission with Occasional Relapses** —
Patients in remission, who have been without symptoms

panic disorder — a psychiatric disorder marked by intense
anxiety and panic as well as
many physical symptoms, such
as: palpitations, shortness of
breath, dizziness, sweating, and
a sense of impending death

**generalized anxiety
disorder** — a psychiatric
disorder marked by unrealistic
worry, apprehension, and
uncertainty as well as physical
symptoms, such as: muscle tension, restlessness, dry mouth,
and frequent urination

*Biofeedback and relaxation
training (see page 41) is an
example of a physiological
coping strategy.*

schizophrenia — a major
psychiatric disorder characterized by disorganization and
fragmentation of thought,
delusions, hallucinations, apathy,
disturbance of language and
communication, and withdrawal
from social interaction

lifetime PTSD — those who
developed PTSD at any time in
their lives

*Chapters four and five detail
current effective treatments
for PTSD.*

Many Japanese survivors (who had functioned well for decades) of the World War II bombing of Kobe had a relapse of PTSD symptoms following the major earthquake of 1995. They reported that the physical sensations (rumbling and tremors of the earth), the enormous death and destruction that surrounded them, and the threat to life of loved ones, recalled long-dormant memories and feelings evoked by the bombing attacks 50 years earlier.

for some time may suddenly relapse and begin to exhibit the full pattern of PTSD symptoms. When this occurs, it is likely that they were recently exposed to some situation that resembled the original traumatic event in a significant way.

3. **Delayed Onset** — In the delayed variant of PTSD, individuals exposed to a traumatic event do not exhibit the PTSD syndrome until months or years later. As with relapse, the immediate precipitant is usually a situation that resembles the original trauma in a significant way; for example, an American Vietnam veteran whose child has been suddenly deployed to the war zone in Afghanistan or Iraq.

Because traumatic stimuli have such power to evoke emotional, behavioral, and physiological reactions, it has been possible to develop treatment and research approaches in which individuals with PTSD are exposed to trauma-related stimuli in a controlled setting. Such treatments (e.g., cognitive-behavioral treatment) have proved to be very effective in ameliorating the symptoms of this disorder. In addition, laboratory research, in which subjects with PTSD are exposed to trauma-related stimuli, has furthered our understanding of the biobehavioral abnormalities associated with this disorder.

Key Concepts for Chapter One:

1. Trauma occurs not just from exposure to a catastrophic event, it also depends on the emotional response of the person exposed to such an event.

2. A person must experience trauma-related symptoms and impairments in everyday functioning for at least a month before diagnostic assessment for PTSD would be appropriate.

3. Prevalence rates for PTSD in the U.S. are about five percent in men and 10 percent in women exposed to catastrophic stress. Worldwide, especially where war and terrorism are common, prevalence is much higher and constitutes a major public health challenge.

4. PTSD symptoms fall into three categories: reexperiencing, avoidant/numbing, and hyperarousal; however, key symptoms have to be evaluated also in terms of persistence and severity of functional impairment following a traumatic event.

5. PTSD sufferers can experience the disorder throughout their lifetime (where symptoms are chronic, severe, and permanent), occasionally (as remissions and relapses typically linked to some exposure that resembles the original trauma), and with a delayed onset (occurring months or years following exposure to a traumatic event).

Chapter Two:
Diagnosing and Assessing PTSD

This chapter answers the following:

▶ **What are the DSM-IV(TR) Diagnostic Criteria for PTSD?** — This section includes a reprint of the DSM-IV(TR) criteria and a discussion of each major criterion.

▶ **How Should Clinicians Approach Initial Patient Interviews?** — This section covers strategies for conducting the initial clinical interview as well as PTSD risk factors to identify early in the assessment process.

▶ **What Tools are Available for Diagnosing PTSD?** — This section presents strategies for conducting a clinical interview, identifying risk factors, and using standard measurements to assist in the PTSD diagnosis.

▶ **How do you Differentiate PTSD from Comorbid and other Disorders?** — This section reviews comorbid disorders and other post-traumatic outcomes as well as their prevalence. It also covers how to differentiate from PTSD both co-existing disorders and other conditions that manifest in a person who has experienced trauma.

What are the DSM-IV(TR) Diagnostic Criteria for PTSD?

To be diagnosed with PTSD, a person must have been exposed to trauma and experience symptoms for at least a month after exposure. Figure 2.1, on page 10, presents the DSM-IV(TR) criteria for PTSD. The following provides detailed discussion and examples for these criteria.

The Traumatic Stress Criterion

The DSM-IV(TR) definition of a traumatic event has two components: exposure to a catastrophic event (the A_1 criterion) and emotional distress because of such exposure (the A_2 criterion).[5]

The A_1 Exposure Criterion

People who meet the DSM-IV(TR) A_1 criterion have been exposed to catastrophic events that involve actual or threatened death or serious injury (e.g., military combat, sexual assault, physical attack, torture, man-made/natural disasters, accidents, incarceration, or exposure to war-zone/urban/domestic violence). Others meeting the A_1 criterion include people not directly endangered, but who witness such events and people who witness the violent aftermath of a catastrophic event (such as dead body parts) but were never personally in danger. Finally, DSM-IV(TR) adds "confronted with" a life-threatening event to the A_1 criterion (e.g., someone learns that a loved one has died during a catastrophic event, but has experienced no personal danger).

> *"Mothers of the Disappeared" are women whose children were arrested by police during the state-sponsored terrorism of the "Dirty War" in Argentina, when the military junta arrested, incarcerated, tortured, and often executed individuals whom they considered subversive. These mothers may or may not have witnessed any more than the arrest of their children. In all cases, however, their children's continued disappearance was a very strong indication that they may have been executed. According to DSM-IV, these mothers have all suffered exposure to an A_1 event, because they have been "confronted with" the probable violent death of their children.*

Figure 2.1   DSM-IV (TR) Diagnostic Criteria for Post-Traumatic Stress Disorder[5]

A. The person has been exposed to a traumatic event in which both of the following were present:

1. The person experienced, witnessed, or was confronted with an event or events that involved actual or threatened death or serious injury, or a threat to the physical integrity of self or others

2. The person's response involved intense fear, helplessness, or horror.

B. The traumatic event is persistently reexperienced in one (or more) of the following ways:

1. Recurrent and intrusive distressing recollections of the event, including images, thoughts, or perceptions

2. Recurrent distressing dreams of the event

3. Acting or feeling as if the traumatic event were recurring (includes a sense of reliving the experience, illusions, hallucinations and dissociative flashback episodes) (see chapter one).

4. Intense psychological distress at exposure to internal or external cues that symbolize or resemble an aspect of the traumatic event

5. *Physiological reactivity*

C. Persistent avoidance of stimuli associated with the trauma and numbing of general responsiveness (not present before the trauma), as indicated by three (or more) of the following:

1. Efforts to avoid thoughts, feelings, or conversations associated with the trauma

2. Efforts to avoid activities, places, or people that arouse recollections of the trauma

3. Inability to recall an important aspect of the trauma

4. Markedly diminished interest or participation in significant activities

5. Feeling of detachment or estrangement from others

6. Restricted range of affect (e.g., unable to have loving feelings)

7. Sense of a foreshortened future (e.g., does not expect to have a career, marriage, children, or a normal life span)

D. Persistent symptoms of increased arousal not present before the trauma, as indicated by two (or more) of the following:

1. Difficulty falling or staying asleep

2. Irritability or outbursts of anger

3. Difficulty concentrating

4. Hypervigilance

5. Exaggerated startle response

E. Duration of the disturbance (symptoms in Criteria B, C, and D) is more than one month.

F. The disturbance causes clinically significant distress or impairment in social, occupation, or other important areas of functioning.

Specify:

    Acute: if duration of symptoms is less than 3 months

    Chronic: if duration of symptoms is 3 months or more

Specify:

    With delayed onset: if onset of symptoms is at least 6 months after the stressor

Reprinted with permission by the American Psychiatric Association: *Diagnostic and Statistical Manual of Mental Disorder, Fourth Edition Text Revision.* Washington DC: American Psychiatric Association, 2000.

hallucination — a compelling perceptual experience of seeing, hearing, or smelling something that is not actually present

physiological reactivity — quickening of the heart rate, blood pressure, and breathing, resulting from exposure to internal or external cues that symbolize or resemble an aspect of the traumatic event

The A₂ Distress Criterion

People are different. Some people exposed to an A_1 event will experience severe psychological distress, characterized in DSM-IV(TR) as "fear, helplessness, or horror"; others will not exhibit such distress, and still others may have a delayed response.

> ▶ **Those who Experience Significant Distress** — Those people who exhibit intensive distress following an A_1 event meet the PTSD A criterion and can be said to have been "traumatized."

> ▶ **Those who do not Experience Significant Distress** — Those who cope with an A_1 event without exhibiting "fear, helplessness, or horror" do not meet the PTSD A_2 criterion, have not been "traumatized," and cannot have PTSD. This scenario often applies to people who are exposed to A_1 events continually because of their professional responsibilities (such as military, police, and emergency medical personnel) who do not meet the A_2 criterion.

Children, especially those six and younger, who lack an adult's capacity for abstract thinking or linguistic expression, may express their emotional reaction (A_2 reaction) behaviorally rather then verbally through developmentally appropriate, non-verbal indicators of psychological distress, such as disorganized or agitated behavior during play.

A_1 events differ considerably in their capacity to evoke psychological distress; suffering injury due to willful, violent, personal intent (as in rape, assault, or torture) is much more distressing than suffering injury from an impersonal accident or natural disaster. This is a major reason why 46 percent of women who have been raped develop PTSD compared to only nine percent of women involved in an accident.[1]

Multiple Traumas

Although people may develop severe PTSD from one horrific event, as with Mary T. (see below), it is not uncommon in clinical practice to see people who have been exposed to many extremely stressful criterion A experiences. Unfortunately, this is common in cases of childhood sexual or physical trauma, domestic violence, urban violence, forced migration, war, state terrorism (e.g., as torture), or state-sponsored genocide. If the events are sequential episodes of the same traumatic stressor (as in child abuse, war, etc.), psychosocial treatment may be successful by focusing on the "worst" episode (see chapter four). If, however, two or more traumatic stressors are quite different in character (e.g., war trauma and childhood sexual abuse), each A criterion experience may have to be addressed separately during psychotherapy.

Although an individual need not have more than one reexperiencing (B), three avoidant/numbing (C), and two hyperarousal (D) symptoms to meet DSM-IV(TR) diagnostic criteria for PTSD (as stated in figure 2.2 on pages 12 through 14), it is not at all unusual for a traumatized person to exhibit most, if not all, B, C, and D symptoms.

The case study of Mary T. (pages 12 through 14) illustrates this scenario.

Figure 2.2   Diagnosing Mary T.: A Case Study

Trauma Event Symptoms — A Criteria

Mary T. was a 27-year-old, happily married woman. One Sunday while driving to church, her car was hit by a large semi-tractor-trailer that had been unable to stop at a red light because of faulty brakes. The truck was exceeding the speed limit, its momentum was great, and the impact of the collision was tremendous. As the truck crashed into the right side of the car, her husband was killed instantly.

Mary was badly bruised but not seriously injured. Instead, she was trapped in the car for several hours before she could be extricated by the rescue squad. During that period, her dead husband was crushed against her. She was covered with his blood. It was a terrifying and horrifying experience. She recalls an overwhelming sense of loss, despair, and rage as she was trapped in the car waiting to be released but not wanting the separation from her husband that would result.

Reexperiencing Symptoms — B Criteria

After release from the emergency room and a six-week convalescence with her sister in a different city, Mary returned home determined to pick up the pieces and go on with her career as a software designer in a prestigious and very successful computer firm. In cases of PTSD, some or all of Mary's reexperiencing symptoms illustrate how the traumatic event remains, sometimes for decades, a dominating psychological experience that retains its power to evoke panic, terror, dread, grief, or despair.

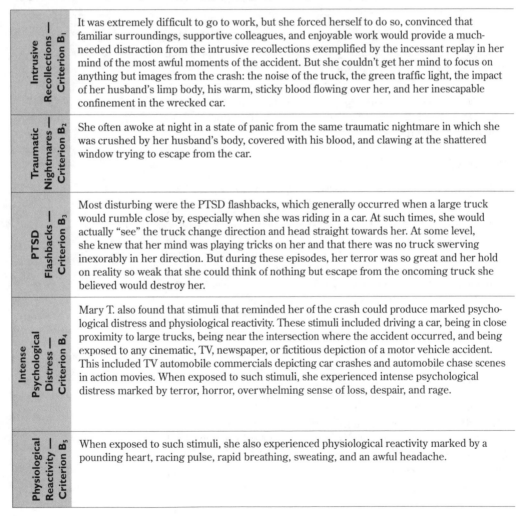

Intrusive Recollections — Criterion B_1	It was extremely difficult to go to work, but she forced herself to do so, convinced that familiar surroundings, supportive colleagues, and enjoyable work would provide a much-needed distraction from the intrusive recollections exemplified by the incessant replay in her mind of the most awful moments of the accident. But she couldn't get her mind to focus on anything but images from the crash: the noise of the truck, the green traffic light, the impact of her husband's limp body, his warm, sticky blood flowing over her, and her inescapable confinement in the wrecked car.
Traumatic Nightmares — Criterion B_2	She often awoke at night in a state of panic from the same traumatic nightmare in which she was crushed by her husband's body, covered with his blood, and clawing at the shattered window trying to escape from the car.
PTSD Flashbacks — Criterion B_3	Most disturbing were the PTSD flashbacks, which generally occurred when a large truck would rumble close by, especially when she was riding in a car. At such times, she would actually "see" the truck change direction and head straight towards her. At some level, she knew that her mind was playing tricks on her and that there was no truck swerving inexorably in her direction. But during these episodes, her terror was so great and her hold on reality so weak that she could think of nothing but escape from the oncoming truck she believed would destroy her.
Intense Psychological Distress — Criterion B_4	Mary T. also found that stimuli that reminded her of the crash could produce marked psychological distress and physiological reactivity. These stimuli included driving a car, being in close proximity to large trucks, being near the intersection where the accident occurred, and being exposed to any cinematic, TV, newspaper, or fictitious depiction of a motor vehicle accident. This included TV automobile commercials depicting car crashes and automobile chase scenes in action movies. When exposed to such stimuli, she experienced intense psychological distress marked by terror, horror, overwhelming sense of loss, despair, and rage.
Physiological Reactivity — Criterion B_5	When exposed to such stimuli, she also experienced physiological reactivity marked by a pounding heart, racing pulse, rapid breathing, sweating, and an awful headache.

Figure 2.2 continued

Avoidant/Numbing Symptoms — C Criterion

Thoughts and memories about the accident evoked such an intense emotional and physiological reaction, that Mary made concerted efforts to avoid thoughts, feelings, or conversations about the trauma as well as activities, places, or people associated with it.

Avoid Thoughts, Feelings or Conversations about the Trauma — Criterion C_1	It was because she didn't want to think about the accident that Mary refused to take legal action against the trucking company that had negligently failed to inspect and repair the truck's faulty brakes. When she found herself involuntarily beginning to think about the accident, she would try to distract herself with music, work, or some other emotionally neutral matter with which she could occupy her mind.
Avoid Activities, Places, or People Associated with the Trauma — Criterion C_2	She avoided riding in a car, traveling on major roadways where she might encounter tractor-trailer trucks, and watching TV or movies for fear that they would contain crash scenes or other images reminiscent of the accident. She even tried to stay awake as long as she could at night to avoid the traumatic nightmares that terrified her three or four times each week.
Inability to Recall an Important Aspect of the Trauma — Criterion C_3	The inability to recall important aspects of the trauma (psychogenic amnesia), which may last for years, differs qualitatively from behavioral avoidance or psychic numbing. Initially, Mary was certain that she had complete recall of the entire event. After all, her problem was not amnesia, but rather that the intrusive recollections and other reexperiencing symptoms were so terribly unbearable that she couldn't work, sleep, or function as she had before the accident. However, after weeks of reviewing and reprocessing the event with her psychotherapist, she began to remember more and more details of the accident. She indeed had experienced an inability to recall an important aspect of the trauma. What she began to recall was even worse than what she had remembered. She began to have a vivid recollection of the initial impact when the nose of the truck plowed through the door, sweeping her husband into her lap. Worst still, she now recalled that he didn't die instantly but lived long enough to gaze at her imploringly, his face contorted by pain, looking at her silently, unable to speak, breathing his last, and begging for help. This was the most unbearable memory of all.
Diminished Interest and Stopped Participating — Criterion C_4	Mary T. felt that she had become a very different person since the accident, and she didn't like the changes she perceived in herself. Whereas previously she had been open, emotional, adventurous, and gregarious, she was now withdrawn, unresponsive, wooden, and solitary. She exhibited diminished interest and stopped participating in the many social, athletic, and church activities in which she had previously been very active.
Detached and Estranged From Others — Criterion C_5	She felt detached and estranged from others, especially from her sister and two closest friends, partially because she was convinced that no one could possibly know or understand how her old self had been irreversibly changed by the accident. It was, therefore, impossible for her to maintain interpersonal relationships as before. She didn't want to be with others and actively resisted their efforts to spend time with her.

Figure 2.2 continued

Restricted Range of Affect — Criterion C₆	She felt numb, wooden, and hollow inside, as if her capacity for emotional experience and expression had been completely anesthetized. This restricted range of affect made it impossible for Mary to enjoy companionship or reciprocate feelings of warmth, friendship, intimacy, or love.
Fore-shortened Future — Criterion C₇	Finally, she felt that her life was over, that she had a foreshortened future with no career, marriage, children, or normal life span to look forward to.

Hyperarousal Symptoms — D Criterion

Mary T. was in a state of constant arousal, agitation, and anxiety. Others perceived her as being jumpy, nervous, easily upset, and having a hair-trigger temper. She had difficulty falling or staying asleep.

Difficulty Falling or Staying Asleep — Criterion D¹	Insomnia occurred either because she couldn't distract her mind from intrusive recollections of the trauma, because she was awakened by traumatic nightmares, or because her high level of physiological overdrive was too much to permit sleep.
Irritability or Outbursts of Anger — Criterion D₂	She exhibited irritability or outbursts of anger that astonished friends who had previously regarded her as an easy-going and resilient individual with a great sense of humor.
Difficulty Concentrating — Criterion D₃	She had difficulty concentrating because her mind was preoccupied with intrusive recollections or because her arousal level was so high that she could not focus on any intellectual task for a sustained period. This was such a problem that she had to take a leave of absence from her job.
Hypervigilance — Criterion D₄	Mary became obsessed with fears about personal safety. The tragic and traumatic accident that had killed her husband made her hypervigilant for the first sign of danger. This was especially noticeable when she was in a car, but it also included being reluctant to go shopping alone, refusing to venture out of her house after dark, and installing an elaborate security system in her home.
An Exaggerated Startle Response — Criterion D₅	Finally, she was extremely jumpy and would exhibit an exaggerated startle response to any unexpected noise. The exquisitely sensitive startle reflex is a well-understood adaptive response to trauma that has been studied extensively in both animal and human research.

Clinically Significant Distress and Impairment — F Criterion

Mary T.'s PTSD caused clinically significant distress and impairment socially (e.g., withdrawal from friends, relationships, and activities), occupationally (e.g., a leave of absence from work because of her inability to function), and in other important areas of functioning. Therefore, she met Functional Impairment (F) Criterion.

Diagnosis: Chronic PTSD

Mary T. has chronic PTSD because her symptoms persisted much longer than three months.

How Should Clinicians Approach Initial Patient Interviews?

In general, PTSD is not a difficult diagnosis to make if the clinician keeps the diagnostic criteria in mind. It is essential, however, that the clinician conduct the diagnostic interview in a manner that acknowledges the patient's worst fears and that provides an environment of sensitivity, safety, and trust. After all, the clinician is asking the PTSD patient to take a tremendous risk and abandon all the avoidance behaviors, protective and other psychological strategies that buffer the patient from the intolerable memories and feelings associated with the traumatic event.

In the case of chronic PTSD, where protective layers have solidified for years or decades, the clinician must be patient and obtain the trauma history at a pace that the patient can tolerate. It is usually helpful to immediately acknowledge to the patient how difficult it must be to answer these questions. It is also helpful for the clinician to encourage the patient to indicate when the interview becomes too upsetting and to back off immediately when the patient communicates this.

By exhibiting clinical behavior that communicates patience, sensitivity, and competence, it is usually possible to obtain a thorough diagnostic assessment from the most anxious, avoidant, and hypervigilant patient.

Since most people who experience trauma do not develop PTSD, understanding who might be at greater risk is important. The factors listed in figure 2.3, on the next page, are associated with greater risk for PTSD.[17, 18] Although this table identifies many pre-traumatic risk factors, they have only modest power as PTSD predictors. A recent meta-analysis indicates that the strongest risk factors were severity ("dose") of the trauma and poor post-traumatic social support.[17]

From the Patient's Perspective

Well, I did it! I sat through two hours with that psychologist. I couldn't believe there were so many questions. I also couldn't believe that so many of them seemed to fit. Right on target about all that's been bothering me. I did pretty well at first. And I didn't mind telling her what a mess I've been. How my nerves are shot. The nightmares. And all the rest. But when she started asking about the accident, I lost it. I just couldn't go on. And I'm getting so upset just thinking about it that I'd better stop right now.

Figure 2.3   Risk Factors for PTSD

Pre-Traumatic

- **Gender** — Women are twice as likely as men to develop PTSD at some point in their lives, partially due to the likelihood of experiencing interpersonal violence (e.g., rape, sexual molestation, parental neglect, childhood sexual/physical abuse).
- **Age** — Adults younger than 25 are most at risk.
- **Education** — Those with less than a college education are more at risk.
- **Childhood Trauma** — Child abuse (including sexual abuse), rape, war, or motor vehicle accidents can increase risk.
- **Childhood Adversity** — Economic deprivation or parental separation/divorce before the child is age 10 can be a factor.
- **Adverse Life Events** — Divorce, loss of job, failure at school, financial problems, or poor physical health can increase risk.
- **Psychiatric Disorders** — Those diagnosed with a childhood conduct disorder (e.g., Attention Deficit Hyperactivity Disorder) or those with any prior psychiatric disorder are most at risk, as are those with a *personality pathology*.
- **Genetics** — Family history of any psychiatric disorder or possible genetic differences in regulating pre-synaptic uptake of serotonin can increase risk.*

personality pathology — maladaptive pattern of relating to other people that severely impairs social functioning and adaptive potential

Traumatic

- **Severity ("dose") of the Trauma** — The greater the magnitude of trauma exposure, the greater the likelihood of developing PTSD.
- **Nature of the Trauma** — Interpersonal violence (e.g., rape, physical attack, torture, war-zone trauma), in which there is a human perpetrator, is much more likely to produce PTSD than an impersonal event (e.g., natural disaster).
- **Betrayal** — When a parent or caregiver on whom the victim is completely dependent perpetrates interpersonal violence, as in childhood sexual abuse, the trauma is more likely to produce PTSD than when the perpetrator is a stranger.
- *Peritraumatic Dissociation* — This symptom, as seen in acute stress disorder (ASD), is more likely to predict the later development of PTSD than if the trauma survivor did not experience dissociative symptoms at the time of the trauma.
- **Participation in Atrocities** — Being either a perpetrator or witness of atrocities has proven to be a risk factor for Vietnam and other military veterans.

peritraumatic dissociation — dissociation during and shortly after the trauma

Post-Traumatic

- **Poor Social Support** — After exposure to trauma, lack of social support is a risk factor for the onset of PTSD.
- **Development of Acute Stress Disorder (ASD)** — ASD is a strong indication of post-traumatic symptom severity and predicts the later development of PTSD among 80 percent of affected individuals (see chapter six).
- **Access to Acute, Post-traumatic Clinical Intervention** — As discussed in chapter six, timely treatment of ASD can prevent the later development of PTSD.

*Recent genetic research has shown that, of the two variants of the gene regulating pre-synaptic uptake of serotonin, the long form appears to be associated with resilience and the short form with vulnerability to stressful events. Individuals who inherited the short form and were exposed to four or more stressful life events were much more likely to develop depression or to attempt suicide.[19] Although this has yet to be tested in PTSD, it does suggest (as have twin studies) that there is a genetic vulnerability to PTSD.[20]

What Tools are Available for Diagnosing PTSD?

Diagnosing PTSD can take several meetings in which the clinician conducts a careful interview, asking questions on risk factors for PTSD and ruling out other possible disorders. Additionally, clinicians may utilize assessment tools, such as structured interviews or *psychometric instruments*. Instruments for assessing exposure to trauma, for diagnosing, and for determining the severity of PTSD symptoms in adults and children are discussed later in this chapter and described in detail in appendices A and B.

psychometric instruments — tests that measure psychological factors, such as personality, intelligence, beliefs, and fears

Using Structured Interviews and Questionnaires

Many structured interviews and questionnaires exist for assessing and diagnosing PTSD. These instruments fall into three overlapping categories:

Appendix A describes instruments designed for adults; Appendix B covers those developed exclusively for children.

1. **Trauma Exposure Scales** determine exposure to a criterion A_1 event by documenting the nature and severity of such overwhelming stressors. General exposure questionnaires inquire about exposure to all possible kinds of catastrophic events, while specific exposure scales may focus on child abuse, domestic violence, rape, combat exposure, or torture.

2. **Diagnostic Instruments** take the form of structured interviews administered by a clinician or lay interviews designed for survey research. These often broad-spectrum instruments inquire about all DSM-IV (TR) diagnoses with a separate specific module dedicated to PTSD diagnostic criteria. Such instruments may also detect comorbid diagnoses.

3. **Symptom Severity Scales** are primarily available for PTSD, usually as self-report questionnaires in which individuals indicate (usually on a four or five point scale) the intensity of a specific PTSD symptom (such as traumatic nightmares).

Within this class of instruments are structured clinical interviews that can be used both as diagnostic instruments and symptom severity scales [e.g., the Clinician Administered PTSD Scale (CAPS)].

In practice, it is usually best to start with a general trauma exposure scale. If the patient reports previous exposure to a criterion A_1 event, one can either inquire in more detail about the specific trauma exposure (e.g., child abuse) or proceed directly to a diagnostic instrument to determine whether PTSD is present. PTSD severity can next be determined with a symptom severity scale or with the Clinician Administered PTSD Scale (CAPS), which is both a diagnostic instrument and symptom severity scale (see appendix A).

A thorough and comprehensive discussion of PTSD assessment can be found in a recent book devoted entirely to this topic.[21]

How do you Differentiate PTSD from Comorbid and Other Disorders?

comorbid disorders — major psychiatric disorders that are present at the same time an individual has full-fledged PTSD

A victim of trauma may suffer from *comorbid* psychiatric disorders in addition to PTSD or their trauma may result in a disorder that is different from PTSD.

Other Axis I Psychiatric Syndromes — Individuals with lifetime PTSD likely meet DSM-IV(TR) diagnostic criteria for at least one other Axis I psychiatric disorder. Indeed, 80 percent of all men and women with lifetime PTSD in the National Comorbidity Study also met criteria for at least one of the following: major depressive disorder, dysthymia, generalized anxiety disorder, simple phobia, social phobia, panic disorder, alcohol abuse/dependence, drug abuse/dependence, or conduct disorder.[1]

Comorbidity is important to keep in mind when conducting a diagnostic assessment or formulating a treatment plan for someone suspected of having PTSD.

Figure 2.4, below, illustrates prevalence rates for comorbid disorders. One reason for such high prevalence of comorbid disorders is the symptom overlap between PTSD and these other Axis I diagnoses.

Figure 2.4   DSM-IV(TR) Disorders Frequently Comorbid with PTSD

Diagnosis	Lifetime Prevalence (%)
Major Depressive Disorder	48
Dysthymia	22
Generalized Anxiety Disorder	16
Simple Phobia	30
Social Phobia	28
Panic Disorder	12.6 vs. 7.3*
Agoraphobia	22.4 vs. 16.1*
Alcohol Abuse/Dependence	51.9 vs. 27.9**
Drug Abuse/Dependence	34.5 vs. 26.9**
Conduct Disorder	43.3 vs. 15.4**

*women > men   **men > women

From the *National Comorbidity Survey*[1]

There is growing evidence that PTSD may not be the only clinically significant consequence of exposure to a catastrophic event. Other types of post-traumatic outcomes discussed should also receive clinician/researcher attention. Furthermore, some people exposed to traumatic stress never exhibit PTSD. Instead, they may develop depression, alcoholism, or some other DSM-IV(TR) disorder.

Medical Disorders — Growing evidence indicates that exposure to catastrophic events is a risk factor for many medical disorders affecting the cardiovascular, gastrointestinal, endocrinological, musculoskeletal, and other bodily systems.[12, 22]

Partial/Subsyndromal PTSD — There is growing interest in people who lack only one or two of the three mandatory DSM-IV(TR) symptoms (see page 6). A number of studies have shown that such individuals have clinically significant, post-traumatic symptoms and functional impairment.[23-25]

Complex PTSD — Prolonged trauma, especially childhood sexual abuse or torture during political incarceration, may produce a clinical syndrome that differs considerably from that seen in PTSD. This syndrome provisionally called, "complex PTSD," features: impulsivity, dissociation, *somatization, affect lability*, interpersonal difficulties, and *pathological changes* in personal identity (dissociative identity disorder in DSM-IV; previously multiple personality disorder in DSM-III).[26]

There is growing evidence that PTSD may not be the only clinically significant consequence of exposure to a catastrophic event. Differentiating PTSD symptoms from other disorders involves considering factors such as:

1. **Affective Disorders** — PTSD patients may exhibit similar symptoms to depression or dysthymia (insomnia, impaired concentration, social withdrawal, and diminished interest in activities). However, affective disorders are more characterized than PTSD by depressed mood, decreased capacity for enjoyment, guilt, weight loss, suicidal thoughts, and a slowing of thoughts and actions (e.g., "psychomotor retardation").

2. **Generalized Anxiety Disorder (GAD)** — Patients with PTSD exhibit irritability, hypervigilance, exaggerated startle response, impaired concentration, insomnia, and autonomic hyperarousal; however, GAD is more likely if there is the presence of: unrealistic worry, muscle tension, restlessness, dry mouth, frequent urination, and a lump in the throat.

3. **Phobias** (e.g., simple phobia, social phobia, and agoraphobia) — Although some patients exhibit both avoidant and arousal behaviors typical of PTSD, perhaps triggered by environmental and/or social stimuli, phobia patients do not exhibit the numbing symptoms seen in PTSD.

4. **Panic Disorder** — Symptoms resemble PTSD because they include many symptoms of autonomic hyperarousal and because panic patients may exhibit dissociation. In contrast to stimulus-driven PTSD symptoms, however, panic attacks are unexpected and occur spontaneously; they are associated with symptoms of choking, numbness, tingling, fear of going crazy, and fear of dying.

5. **Chemical Abuse/Dependency** — Often seen in PTSD patients as a comorbid diagnosis, there are no symptoms concerning use and misuse of alcohol or drugs that are part of the PTSD diagnostic criteria.

somatization — the expression of emotional distress through physical symptoms such as peptic ulcer, asthma, or chronic pain

affect lability — rapid and unpredictable shifts in mood state

pathological changes — changes resulting in an abnormal condition that prevents proper psychological functioning

Phobia patients become aroused only when they believe they will be exposed to the feared stimulus or situation. PTSD patients, on the other hand, are perpetually in a state of hyperarousal.

Key Concepts for Chapter Two:

1. DSM-IV (TR) criteria for PTSD require that, for at least a month after being exposed to a traumatic event, a person suffers intense emotional responses, persistently re-experiences elements of the event, regularly avoids stimuli associated with the trauma, becomes somewhat "numb," and suffers increased arousal.

2. PTSD symptoms must cause significant distress or impairment in social, occupational, or other important areas of functioning.

3. Diagnosis and assessment must be conducted in an environment of sensitivity, safety, and trust for the patient to be able to recount information about the traumatic event and its aftermath.

4. Those who may be more likely to develop PTSD following exposure to a traumatic event are women, young adults, those with a personal or family history of psychiatric disorders, and people who have experienced childhood trauma/adversity or adverse life events as adults.

5. The severity and nature of the trauma can significantly impact one's risk of developing PTSD.

6. Onset of PTSD following exposure to a traumatic event is more likely if the person has developed (and especially not been treated for) acute stress disorder as well as if the person lacks social support.

7. There are a variety of tools available for assessing and diagnosing PTSD, including trauma exposure scales, diagnostic instruments, and symptom severity scales.

8. Mental health disorders typically comorbid with PTSD are major depressive disorder, dysthymia, other anxiety disorders, substance abuse, and conduct disorder. Additionally, PTSD sufferers tend to also experience a variety of medical disorders.

Chapter Three:
Global Treatment Issues for PTSD

This chapter answers the following:

▶ **What are the Timing and Priority Issues Related to Treatment?** — This section covers issues surrounding the timing of when patients seek treatment as well as priorities in PTSD treatment (e.g., psychiatric emergency, alcohol or drug abuse/ dependence, comorbidity, and situational factors).

▶ **What General Considerations Exist for Choosing a Specific Treatment Option?** — This section provides an overview of treatment considerations, such as combining treatments, comorbid disorders, and complex PTSD.

▶ **What PTSD Treatment-Focus Issues Exist?** — This section covers decision making on trauma vs. supportive therapy, using combined treatments, and other issues.

▶ **What are the Major Personal Issues for Clinicians Treating Those with PTSD?** — This section discusses therapeutic neutrality, advocacy, secondary traumatization, countertransference, and clinician self-care.

Aﬀﬂ FTER determining that a patient requesting treatment has PTSD, there are a number of questions clinicians need to address. In most respects, these questions are no different than with other psychiatric disorders, although the presence of PTSD sometimes raises questions about treatment timing priorities, focus, and approach.

What are the Timing and Priority Issues Related to Treatment?

For clinicians, global treatment issues often begin with answering the question, "Why seek help now?" and proceed to determining what issues or situations may delay or alter a typical PTSD treatment approach.

Timing Issues for Seeking Treatment

When people complain about the recent onset of reexperiencing, avoidant/numbing, or hyperarousal symptoms, it is usually pretty obvious why they are seeking treatment at this time and that PTSD is the first (and possibly only) order of business. On the other hand, when people who have had chronic PTSD for many years suddenly request treatment, it is usually because something has changed abruptly in their lives. This change has disrupted their equilibrium in terms of coping both with PTSD symptoms and the demands of family, friends, work, and society.

Examples of obvious reasons for someone with chronic PTSD to seek treatment at a given time include:

▶ *A woman, who was raped many years ago, was recently sexually harassed or threatened.*

▶ *A combat veteran, who now works as a police officer, has had his partner seriously wounded in a gunfight or thought he might be killed himself in the same encounter.*

Sometimes the precipitant is obvious; however, at other times, the clinician must take a careful history to identify the recent precipitant. For example:

▶ A Red Cross disaster worker complains of traumatic nightmares related to an event s/he had not thought about for a long time. It is likely that certain specific details of a recent disaster reactivated memories of a similar event in the past, about which there remain intense, unresolved emotional feelings.

▶ A woman who has successfully dealt with the emotional consequences of her own childhood sexual abuse begins having intrusive recollections of this traumatic experience when her adolescent daughter begins dating or becomes sexually active.

▶ A military veteran may experience a reexacerbation of symptoms when television coverage focuses on new military offensives (e.g., Iraq, Persian Gulf, Bosnia, Somalia, etc.) or when a child is called up for military duty.

▶ For older veterans, the death of an adult child (even by natural causes such as cancer) may reactivate survival guilt about having outlived friends at Normandy Beach or in Vietnam.

well encapsulated — psychological buffers that prevent a person from experiencing current distress from a previous traumatic event

Some trauma-related stimuli can be heavily disguised. Take the example of a successful business woman with a *well-encapsulated* sexual trauma history that has caused no previous emotional difficulty. She may suddenly develop PTSD symptoms when her professional advancement seems unfairly and consistently blocked by hostile or oppressive male superiors, leaving her feeling powerless. Although the precipitating stressor is in the workplace, her nightmares are inexplicably (to her) about the sexual abuse she suffered decades earlier.

From the Patient's Perspective

I've got to hand it to her. She asked about everything. About how depressed I've been. About how hard this has been on my relationships. And about possible problems that never would have occurred to me, like drinking and such. But at the end, she decided, and I agreed, that the major problem was the PTSD and that we really needed to consider how this accident has turned my life upside down.

Priority Issues for Treatment

In the examples on the previous page, PTSD is clearly the first order of business, and the clinician must develop a treatment plan that addresses both the current precipitant as well as unresolved past traumatic issues that have become central to the current clinical problem. Sometimes, however, PTSD may not be the first order of business because other clinical issues must take priority before PTSD treatment can be initiated. Common reasons for delaying PTSD treatment include the existence of:

- A psychiatric emergency (the patient is suicidal, homicidal, or otherwise so out of control that they need the safety, structure, and control of an inpatient hospital setting)
- Serious alcohol or drug abuse/dependence or comorbid disorder that must be treated before PTSD
- A marital/familial/workplace crisis that demands immediate attention

In a psychiatric emergency, where the patient must be hospitalized without delay, a discharge plan can be developed that will implement PTSD treatment along with other necessary measures when these patients are ready to leave the hospital.

What General Considerations Exist for Choosing a Specific Treatment Option?

When creating a treatment plan for someone with PTSD, there are a number of factors to consider, including:

- **Combined Treatment** — To provide the best possible care for patients, clinicians often combine different therapies (e.g., individual therapy and medication).
- **Treatment of Comorbid Disorders** — Treatments may need to be chosen that address multiple disorders at the same time.
- **Treating "Complex PTSD"** — For those who experienced severe trauma, a new clinical syndrome has been proposed, perhaps demanding a longer-term treatment plan.[26, 27]
- **Cross-Cultural Considerations** — Clinicians need to be sensitive to cultural differences in PTSD assessment and treatment.
- **Recovered Memories** — Controversy exists over whether or not previously forgotten traumatic memories can be recovered many years later as well as how these memories should be addressed by clinicians.
- **Safety** — It is emotionally dangerous for PTSD patients to relinquish the cognitive, emotional, and behavioral avoidant strategies they use to cope with intolerable intrusive recollections and arousal symptoms.

Clinicians must establish an atmosphere of trust and safety, thereby "earning the right to gain access" to carefully guarded traumatic material.[28]

What PTSD Treatment-Focus Issues Exist?

Many treatments for PTSD encourage the patient to specifically remember and focus on the experienced trauma (trauma-focus treatment). Others encourage the patient to increase coping skills for current here-and-now stressors to improve daily functioning and decrease PTSD symptoms (supportive therapy). Sometimes, therapy is combined with medication. And sometimes, comorbid disorders must be treated before PTSD treatment can begin.

Trauma Focus

psychodynamic approaches — therapeutic approaches that focus on unconscious and conscious motivations and drives

cognitive-behavioral approaches — therapeutic approaches that focus on patterns of reinforcement, learning and conditioning models, and correcting erroneous cognitions

Trauma focus therapy uses the in-depth exploration of traumatic material to facilitate healing. As described in chapter four, pages 36 through 46, it can be conducted in individual or group contexts with techniques that vary from *psychodynamic* to *cognitive-behavioral* (CBT) *approaches.*[28, 29] The goal of trauma focus therapy is for patients to take control of their lives by gaining authority over traumatic memories.

Trauma Focus vs. Supportive Therapy

For more information on CBT treatment approaches, see pages 36 through 42.

Trauma focus treatment may not be beneficial for everyone. Most research data on trauma focus treatments apply only to those patients who have agreed to undergo such treatment. Although scientific evidence shows that CBT-focused treatment has proven to be the most effective treatment to date (see below), some patients have absolutely no wish to revisit traumatic material because they:

► Want to put the past behind them
► Fear that they cannot tolerate the intrusive and arousal symptoms exacerbated by such memories

When patients' lives remain dangerous because of physical/sexual abuse, domestic violence, war, or an otherwise unsafe environment, they cannot benefit from trauma focus work. Supportive therapy and medication treatment (see chapter four) are better options than trauma focus therapy until personal safety can be attained.

Supportive PTSD treatments encourage skill-building and problem solving for current issues in the patient's life as an avenue for increasing adaptive functioning and regaining a sense of control. Supportive treatments that deliberately avoid traumatic material may be beneficial for some with PTSD, although their efficacy has yet to be demonstrated. Currently, there are no guidelines for determining which patients will most likely benefit from one therapy over the other.

There are a number of different PTSD treatments, many of which can be used in combination. Comprehensive practice guidelines for PTSD treatment have been developed by the International Society for Traumatic Stress Studies, the American Psychiatric Association, and jointly by the U.S. Department of Defense and Veterans Affairs.[31-33]

These treatments are:

▶ **Psychoeducational approaches,** in which patients learn about common symptoms and experiences suffered by those with PTSD

▶ **Individual Psychotherapies,** which focus on PTSD symptoms through various methods, such as cognitive-behavioral therapy (CBT); eye-movement desensitization reprocessing (EMDR), or psychodynamic psychotherapy

▶ **Group Therapies,** in which trauma survivors learn about PTSD and help each other with the aid of a professional clinician

▶ **Treatments for children** that are age-appropriate interventions, often extrapolated from adult treatment methods

▶ **Other treatments** that have not been systematically tested with PTSD patients, such as couples/family therapy, hypnosis, and social rehabilitative therapies

Combined Treatment

Clinicians often combine treatment methods. For example, medication combined with individual psychotherapy treatment may not only ameliorate psychobiological abnormalities associated with PTSD, but also sufficiently reduce symptoms so patients can participate in trauma focus treatment. Some patients receive individual treatment plus marital, family, or group therapy, while others may take medication as well.

Unfortunately, there are no published studies in which combined therapy is compared with either psychotherapy or pharmacotherapy alone. Preliminary analysis of an ongoing study suggests that, among medication partial responders, positive treatment results were greatly enhanced when prolonged exposure (see pages 37–38) was combined with medication.[34]

When considering combined treatment, however, it is important to be selective and to recognize that many patients do not need more than one form of treatment at any one time.[35] Good clinical practice requires introducing only one therapeutic approach at a time, carefully gauging its effectiveness before combining with another.

Chapter four presents detailed information on psychological treatment approaches for PTSD.

Pharmacotherapy, in which patients receive medications to help manage PTSD symptoms, is covered in detail in chapter four.

Treatment of Comorbid Disorders

Most patients with PTSD will have at least one comorbid psychiatric disorder; therefore, the treatment approach should seek to ameliorate both PTSD and comorbid disorders.

Alcohol or Drug Abuse/Dependence

It appears that treatments that address comorbid alcohol/drug abuse/dependence and PTSD simultaneously are preferable to addressing each problem separately. Unfortunately, simultaneous treatments are generally untested, not widely available, and challenging as each disorder exacerbates the other.[36]

It is a waste of time to initiate PTSD treatment when someone is too caught up in the addiction intoxication/withdrawal cycle to participate meaningfully in any psychotherapeutic initiative. Many clinicians refuse to work with patients if they come to appointments intoxicated or if they are unable to work in psychotherapy because of their alcohol or drug abuse/dependency. If the chemical abuse/dependency is severely disruptive, they may need to undergo inpatient detoxification and post-detoxification alcohol or drug rehabilitation (that often includes a commitment to attend Alcoholics Anonymous or Narcotics Anonymous meetings).

Clinicians must prepare and protect their patients from the fantasy that once sobriety has been achieved, all will be well. Sadly, the opposite is sometimes the case for patients with PTSD. This is because alcohol and (prescription or illicit) drug abuse often serve to blunt or numb intolerable PTSD reexperiencing or hyperarousal symptoms. During the acute withdrawal period within the first few days of detoxification, previous alcohol/drug-suppressed PTSD symptoms come raging to the forefront of conscious awareness.[36] More importantly, the PTSD patient who has successfully undergone detoxification is now suddenly thrust into the world without this protection. This is why simultaneous treatment is so important.

Co-Existing Psychiatric Disorders

Eighty percent of people who ever suffer PTSD have at least one other psychiatric disorder during their lives. As a result, clinicians must consider whether to treat comorbid disorders before or along with PTSD. Sometimes the severity of the comorbid disorder demands initial attention. For example, a severely depressed individual (with comorbid PTSD) may need aggressive depression treatment, such as medication, before PTSD treatment can be considered. The same holds true for people with an immobilizing panic disorder, individuals whose eating disorder has seriously compromised their health, or persons with other psychiatric problems that are currently more incapacitating or potentially dangerous than the PTSD.

Similarly, some family, vocational, or environmental situations may require intervention before addressing PTSD. For example:

▶ A woman whose PTSD is the result of ongoing domestic violence is a poor candidate for psychotherapy, especially CBT, as long as she remains in an abusive relationship.

Here, the first order of business is providing a safe and secure living situation (e.g., a battered women's shelter or safe house).

▶ A marriage on the brink of collapse because of one member's PTSD symptoms needs couples therapy before starting individual therapy for the PTSD sufferer.

▶ An employee working in conditions perceived to be unsafe has PTSD symptoms continually stirred up by workplace conditions. The immediate challenge is to reduce incapacitating anxiety before PTSD treatment can begin. This could be accomplished by assignment to another tour of duty, by changes in the working environment, or by a medical/psychiatric leave of absence.

"Complex PTSD"

Many clinicians who work with victims of prolonged trauma, such as incest and torture, argue that these patients suffer from a clinical syndrome named "Complex PTSD" (see chapter two), which is not adequately characterized by the current PTSD construct.[26] The non-PTSD symptoms that comprise complex PTSD include:

▶ **Behavioral difficulties** (e.g., impulsivity, aggression, sexual acting out, eating disorders, alcohol/drug abuse, and self-destructive actions)

▶ **Emotional difficulties** (e.g., affective lability, rage, depression, and panic)

▶ **Cognitive difficulties** (e.g., *fragmented thoughts*, dissociation, and *amnesia)*

▶ **Somatization** (e.g., physical symptoms and pain)

▶ **Identity confusion** (previously called multiple personalities)

The validity of complex PTSD as a unique diagnostic entity is controversial. Many PTSD experts point out that there is very little scientific support for this diagnosis and that the vast majority of patients with complex PTSD have already met diagnostic criteria for PTSD. They also often meet diagnostic criteria for borderline personality disorder, somatization disorder, and dissociative identity disorder.[26] This controversy has, so far, excluded complex PTSD from the DSM-IV (TR).

Proponents of the complex PTSD construct suggest that treatment for complex PTSD usually requires long-term individual and group therapies focusing on family function, vocational rehabilitation, social skills training, and alcohol/drug rehabilitation.[26] Dialectical behavior therapy (see page 42) has also been proposed as an effective treatment for complex PTSD.[37]

Military personnel in a war zone, who do not make a timely recovery from acute stress reactions (see chapter six), may need to be removed to the safety of a rear echelon medical unit where they can receive appropriate intervention.

fragmented thoughts — the inability to sustain continuity and coherence in one's cognitive processes

amnesia — mental syndrome characterized by partial or complete memory loss

Several resources offer detailed discussions of culturally sensitive treatment for trauma survivors.[38–40]

calor — a stress-related syndrome observed among Salvadoran women described as a surge of intense heat that may rapidly spread throughout the entire body for a few moments or for several days

ataques de nervios — a common symptom of distress among Hispanic American groups involving anxiety, uncontrollable shouting and crying, trembling, heart palpitations, difficulty breathing, dizziness, fainting spells, and dissociative symptoms (e.g., amnesia and alteration of consciousness)

A recently published, balanced review of recovered memories is in **Post-traumatic Stress Disorder: Malady or Myth?** by C.R. Brewin (2003).[47]

Cross-Cultural Considerations

PTSD has been criticized from a cross-cultural perspective as a Euroamerican construct that fails to take into account culture-specific causes of stress that might be seen in trauma survivors from more traditional cultures. Some symptoms fall outside strict DSM-IV (TR) diagnostic criteria but appear to be dramatic indications of clinically significant post-traumatic distress in their own right.[41] For example, in Latin America, people are diagnosed with *"calor"* and *"ataques de nervios."*

Clinicians need to be attuned to such culture-specific idioms of distress so that they can identify post-traumatic distress when appropriate. It is also essential that, having made the diagnosis, clinicians initiate a culturally sensitive variant of PTSD treatment that will work. For example, an egalitarian approach to family therapy is incomprehensible in some cultures where the father holds a position of authority that cannot be challenged. Likewise, clinicians pressuring for overt discussion of sexual trauma by unmarried Islamic women in group therapy fail to recognize the shameful and potentially socially disastrous consequences of such disclosure.

Recovered Memories

Controversy exists as to whether or not a person can recover trauma memories many years after the trauma occurred.[42] Adults who had been sexually assaulted as children sometimes have no memories of these childhood assaults.[43] Sometimes, such missing traumatic memories later become accessible so that patients then recall traumatic childhood events such as father-daughter incest.[42, 44]

In some cases, recovered memories have been authenticated by external sources whereas in other cases, there is no proof regarding the veracity of the alleged sexual contact.[45, 46] Although there is little rigorous research on this question, it has been suggested that most "recovered" memories have been triggered spontaneously by later life events that resembled the initial trauma; contrary to assertions by some that participation in psychotherapy causes such memories to be "recovered."[42, 48, 49]

Some patients who claim to have regained traumatic memories of this nature have confronted parents whom they now regard as perpetrators of childhood sexual trauma, sometimes taking parents to court for alleged abuses. Sometimes the accused parents vehemently deny that such events ever occurred and maintain that these "traumatic memories" are really emblematic of a "false memory syndrome" manufactured in the course of therapy.[42, 46]

Researchers generally agree that:[42-53]

> Memory, especially childhood memory, is fallible but not necessarily incorrect.

> Documented traumatic events are sometimes forgotten.

> There is adequate proof of a few cases in which forgotten traumatic memories were later "recovered," but it is not known whether this is an extremely rare or frequent event.

Though this issue remains controversial, there is general agreement that clinicians should convey the fallibility of memories and avoid aggressive techniques such as suggesting that patients' symptoms indicate a traumatic experience for which no recollection exists.[42]

Clinicians need to familiarize themselves with the complexity, fallibility, and reconstructive nature of human memory.[42]

What are the Major Personal Issues for Clinicians Treating Those with PTSD?

Clinicians treating individuals with PTSD must deal with how the patient's reports of human suffering impact the clinician personally. Specific issues to note include:

> Therapeutic neutrality vs. advocacy

> *Secondary traumatization*

> *Countertransference*

> Clinician self-care

Therapeutic Neutrality vs. Advocacy

Trauma work challenges the traditional psychotherapeutic principle of clinician *neutrality* because so many people seeking help have suffered from abusive violence, state-sponsored terrorism, or other man-made catastrophes. It is only natural that clinicians' feelings about such injustices are mobilized and channeled into advocacy activities to prevent such human suffering in the future. However, advocacy can undermine therapy.[54] For example, the clinician should never assume the role of rescuer for a specific patient. When a clinician intervenes directly to confront a problem that the patient seems unable to address, it implies that the patient cannot cope with problems without assistance. The more the clinician's words and deeds suggest that the patient is helpless, the more disempowered the patient becomes. Such clinician behavior perpetuates patient beliefs about being personally incompetent and that the world is overwhelming.

In contrast, clinicians can and should act as advocates for patients in obtaining services requiring a professional referral.

secondary traumatization — feelings, personal distress, and symptoms sometimes evoked in people who live with an individual with PTSD

countertransference — the clinician's psychological reaction to something the patient said or did

neutrality — a psychoanalytic technique by which clinicians reveal as little of themselves as possible so that thoughts, memories, and feelings generated during therapy come from the patient's intrapsychic processes rather than from an interpersonal relationship between patient and clinician

Such advocacy might include dealing with local, state, or federal agencies to gain access to community support or victim assistance programs.

Secondary Traumatization

Working with patients who have suffered trauma is difficult. Patients' powerful stories often generate intense emotions within clinicians who may despair because they are powerless to protect patients (especially children) or feel guilty that they were not personally exposed to such horrors.

Secondary traumatization can cause severe personal distress among clinicians and can impair their professional judgment and performance so that their therapeutic efforts become unhelpful or even detrimental to their patients.[55, 56]

Secondary traumatization can produce a number of inappropriate behaviors that compromise therapy or may even disturb the clinician on a personal level, such as engaging in ill-advised rescue attempts or becoming personally involved in the patient's daily life.[54]

Clinicians may become so overwhelmed by the traumatic experiences reported by their patients that they have intrusive recollections and nightmares about such material, which in turn activate avoidant/numbing behavior, guilt, feelings of powerlessness, rescue fantasies, doubting, denial, intellectualization, constricted affect, dissociation, minimization, or avoidance of traumatic material. This process has been called "vicarious traumatization" or "compassion fatigue."[55, 56]

Countertransference

A variety of credible resources address countertransference in the context of PTSD.[54, 57, 58]

Countertransference, a psychoanalytic term, refers to personal memories and feelings elicited from the clinician by the patient in the course of therapy. Whereas secondary traumatization refers to a psychological response that might occur among clinicians who have never experienced trauma, countertransference applies to situations in which patient recollections trigger intrusive recollections in the clinicians of personal traumatic or other significant experiences.

Countertransference most likely occurs when the similarities between patient and clinician experiences are sufficient to trigger the clinician's intrusive recollections, avoidant/numbing, or hyperarousal symptoms as well as other intrapsychic and interpersonal issues.

Since more than half of all American men and women will be exposed to at least one traumatic event during their lives, it is likely that many mental health professionals will also have been traumatized — among whom, some will undoubtedly have developed PTSD.[1]

An important variation on this theme is the countertransference that occurs when clinicians themselves are attempting to cope with the same catastrophic stresses as their patients. For example, clinicians working in a war-zone or natural disaster area are also personally affected by the catastrophic stresses for which their patients seek treatment. Under such circumstances, it is suggested that clinicians seek support, supervision, and possibly treatment for their own post-traumatic distress if they expect to be able to help others.

Clinician Self-Care

Whether due to *vicarious traumatization* or countertransference, disturbing feelings and thoughts can impair both the personal mental health and the professional performance of clinicians treating individuals with PTSD. Clinicians may find themselves trapped in a vicious cycle in which the more symptomatic, maladaptive, and ineffective they become, the more they minimize this state of affairs and plunge themselves into their work. Unfortunately, under such circumstances clinicians most desperately need (but are unlikely to seek) colleague supervision or assistance.

vicarious traumatization — feelings, personal distress, and symptoms that are sometimes evoked in clinicians working with PTSD patients

Recognizing these occupational hazards or personal difficulties is only the first step. Clinicians must make a conscious, sustained, and systematic effort to prevent or remedy vicarious traumatization or countertransference. This can be accomplished through professional and personal self-care activities, such as:[59, 60]

- ▶ Having regular supervision
- ▶ Developing a supportive environment at work
- ▶ Placing limits on one's case load — especially with respect to the number of trauma cases
- ▶ Maintaining boundaries between personal and professional activities
- ▶ Prioritizing personal, marital, and family commitments in relation to professional commitments
- ▶ Engaging in regular exercise, hobbies, friendships, emotional enrichment, artistic endeavors, and spiritual pursuits

Key Concepts for Chapter Three:

1. It is important for clinicians to take a careful history to determine what causes a patient to seek help for chronic PTSD symptoms at a particular time. The timing usually relates to some abrupt change in the patient's life that has disrupted their ability to cope with both the symptoms and daily demands.

2. Clinicians may need to address psychiatric emergencies, substance abuse, or a marital/familial/ workplace crisis prior to initiating treatment for PTSD.

3. Determining the best treatment approach for a patient with PTSD involves consideration of combined treatments, comorbidity, cross-cultural differences in how symptoms are expressed and dealt with, controversial recovered memories, and the patient's emotional safety as well as whether or not a longer, more comprehensive treatment plan should be considered for those who might have "Complex PTSD."

4. Trauma-focused therapy explores the memories of the trauma in-depth to facilitate healing and uses techniques that range from psychodynamic to cognitive behavioral.

5. Supportive therapy focuses on building coping skills and solving problems to enhance functioning and regain a sense of control over one's life.

6. Although untested, simultaneously treating comorbid alcohol and substance abuse/dependence with PTSD appears to be preferable as each disorder exacerbates the other.

7. Patient reports of human suffering and catastrophe can impact clinicians in ways that compromise their therapeutic neutrality, cause them to suffer guilt and feelings of powerlessness that can lead to inappropriate behaviors, or invoke personally painful memories or unresolved feelings (countertransference).

8. Clinicians should attend to their own professional and personal care by creating a supportive work environment with regular supervision, establishing personal boundaries, and limiting case load to maintain a healthy personal/professional balance.

Chapter Four:
Psychological Treatments for PTSD

This chapter answers the following:

▶ **What Specific Psychological Treatments are Available for Adults with PTSD?** — This section reviews the treatment approach and effectiveness of psychoeducation, individual psychotherapy, and group therapy for adult patients with PTSD.

▶ **What Psychological Treatments are Available for Children and Adolescents with PTSD?** — This section covers the treatment approaches used specifically for children and adolescents with PTSD.

What Specific Psychological Treatments are Available for Adults with PTSD?

THERE are many treatments for PTSD, all of which share the general stages and focus of treatment issues discussed in chapter three. Treatments generally fall into three categories:

In this chapter, efficacy research results are covered immediately following the discussion of the approach for each individual therapy. General efficacy information appears with the general overview of each category of treatment.

1. **Psychoeducation** — Designed to help patients understand the nature of PTSD and its impact on their lives

2. **Individual Psychotherapy** — Geared to treat specific symptoms of PTSD through, typically, one of three approaches: cognitive behavioral therapy (CBT), eye movement desensitization reprocessing (EMDR), or psychodynamic psychotherapy (see pages 36 through 44)

3. **Group Therapy** — Structured to treat PTSD in a group setting that promotes a connection among members through shared experiences, which can foster adaptive coping strategies, reduce symptoms, and/or help patients derive meaning from the traumatic experience (see pages 44 through 46).

Psychoeducation

It is relatively easy to move from a comprehensive diagnostic assessment (see chapter two) into a psychoeducational phase of treatment by showing patients how their various reexperiencing, avoidant/numbing, and arousal symptoms fit into a coherent syndrome. Patients need to understand that they are not losing their minds (as many of them genuinely fear to be the case); that their constellation of symptoms has a specific name; and that many other people have suffered in a similar way after exposure to catastrophic stress.

There has been no systematic evaluation of psychoeducation as a stand-alone PTSD treatment. However, there is a strong consensus among clinicians that it is a very important component of any therapeutic approach. In fact, most cognitive-behavioral treatments have a specific psychoeducational component during early treatment sessions.

Psychoeducation may also be especially useful as a societal and community intervention utilizing the mass media to promote resilience and ameliorate distress for the population at large following terrorism or mass casualties (see chapter six).[62]

Psychoeducation to Initiate Therapeutic Activity

The benefits of psychoeducational intervention make it a very powerful and productive way to help patients:

▶ **Achieve Normalization** — Just telling people that the nature of their post-traumatic emotional disturbance is no different than the experience of millions of men, women, and children exposed to similar stresses engenders a profound sense of relief in most people.

▶ **Remove Self-Blame and Self-Doubt** — Telling patients that PTSD is fundamentally about being in the wrong place at the wrong time, and being overwhelmed by a stressor with which no one could have been expected to cope, is a powerful message that most patients can hear readily. It is an important message that helps remove self-blame and self-doubt because most humans do not face these overwhelming events as they would have wished, despite tales of heroes and heroines glorified throughout history.

▶ **Correct Misunderstandings** — Another important benefit of psychoeducation is that the PTSD model helps people understand disturbing behavior that they may have interpreted erroneously. For example, a wife who blames herself for the sexual and emotional withdrawal of her spouse will learn that this is not a personal rejection but rather the expression of her husband's PTSD avoidant/numbing symptoms due to a traumatic event; reframing the problem can focus treatment and often save a marriage before things deteriorate beyond repair.

▶ **Enhance Clinician Credibility** — The final advantage of psychoeducation is that it quickly lets patients know that the clinician understands their problem at its most fundamental level. It is a rapid and effective communication that the clinician deserves trust and is qualified to treat them, helping them make sense of their disturbing and disruptive symptoms.

Psychoeducation through Peer Counseling

One type of psychoeducation, peer counseling, is a powerful group process for PTSD sufferers similar to Alcoholics Anonymous. Peer counseling provides a context of peer support within which participants can take control of their lives by seeking more effective ways to cope with their PTSD symptoms.

Another benefit of peer counseling is that there is no authority figure such as a doctoral-level clinician. Instead, everyone is an equal authority based on his or her own personal experience. Participants are simultaneously patients and clinicians, able to give and receive assistance to one another through honest disclosure and genuine response in the context of absolute trust and confidentiality.

Rape crisis centers and battered women's shelters use peer counseling, as counselors have survived their own sexual trauma and/or domestic violence, found meaning in their suffering, and transformed their personal suffering into knowledge that they use to help others cope with similar experiences. It is reaffirming to know that others have been able to pick up the pieces of their shattered lives and move on to a future that is gratifying and productive.

Since peer counseling is a consumer-driven approach that excludes professional clinicians, it does not lend itself to scientific research protocols in which some patients receive active treatment while others do not. It is clear that people who continue to participate in peer counseling do so because they find the format and support beneficial.

From the Patient's Perspective

Had my fifth session of exposure treatment today. It's hard to admit how scared I was at first. After all, Dr. Owen wanted me to imagine I was back in the car and to go through the whole accident detail by detail. I was terrified and sure that I'd fall apart. But, she was patient. Didn't rush me. And backed off when I started to lose it. Before I knew it, I could really let myself begin to remember what happened. And the more I did it, the easier it got, and the less upset I became.

I'm not there yet. It's still very painful to keep bringing back all that stuff about the accident. But I am getting stronger, and I have another five sessions to go.

Individual Psychotherapies

Clinicians primarily use three different types of individual psychotherapy to treat PTSD:

1. **Cognitive Behavioral Therapy (CBT)** — Based on principals of learning theory and cognitive psychology

2. **Eye Movement Desensitization Reprocessing (EMDR)** — Based on the theory that rapid eye movements reprogram the brain's processing of traumatic memories

3. **Psychodynamic Psychotherapy** — Based on the theory that symptoms of PTSD result from repressed memories of the traumatic event and that the patient's insight into those memories and their impact on symptoms will help restore psychological balance

These therapies can be used in combination and focus on PTSD symptoms through various methods.

Cognitive Behavioral Therapy (CBT)

There are more published well-controlled studies on CBT than on any other PTSD treatment. Furthermore, the magnitude of treatment effects appears greater with CBT than with any other treatment. Two comprehensive reviews are cognitive-behavioral treatment section of Practice Guidelines for PTSD (pp. 60–83) and the VA/DoD Clinical Practice Guidelines for the Management of Post-Traumatic Stress.[33, 61]

Given the fact that PTSD develops when exposure to an overwhelming stimulus (the criterion A_1 event) elicits a profound emotional reaction (the criterion A_2 response), it is understandable why learning and conditioning models have provided such a powerful conceptual approach to PTSD. The sudden, intense anxiety experienced by Mary T. in response to the sight or sound of a large tractor-trailer truck is an excellent example of fear conditioning. Here, the traumatic stimulus (the truck) automatically evokes the post-traumatic emotional response (fear, helplessness, and horror). The intensity of this emotional reaction provokes avoidant behaviors that will reduce the emotional impact of such a stimulus. Successful reduction of intrusion/hyperarousal symptoms will increase the likelihood that avoidant behaviors will be repeated in the future because of their protective value.

From a cognitive psychological perspective, trauma exposure is thought to evoke erroneous automatic thoughts about the environment (as dangerous and threatening) and about oneself (as helpless and incompetent). CBT directly confronts such PTSD-related distortions in thinking.

Various CBT approaches seek to attack these conditioned responses and automatic thoughts with different techniques. The ultimate goal is to normalize the abnormal feelings, thoughts, and behaviors exhibited by individuals with PTSD. CBT has proven to be the best treatment for PTSD in the current published literature; CBT techniques are typically used in combination with one another. Figure 4.1, on the following page, provides an at-a-glance introduction to CBT techniques.

Figure 4.1   Cognitive Behavioral Techniques Used in PTSD Treatment[64-66]

CBT Technique	Treatment Focus
Prolonged Exposure (PE) Therapy	Disconnecting the overwhelming sense of fear from trauma memories
Cognitive Therapy	Relearning thoughts and beliefs generated from the traumatic event, which impede current coping skills
Cognitive Processing Therapy (CPT)	Understanding both the emotional and cognitive consequences of trauma exposure
Stress Inoculation Training (SIT)	Anxiety management to increase coping skills for current situations
Interapy	Exposure and cognitive restructuring through a protocol-driven CBT treatment accessed via the Internet
Imagery Rehearsal Therapy	Changing disturbing traumatic nightmares by rehearsing a "new dream"
Biofeedback and Relaxation Training	Anxiety management to help patients master overwhelming anxiety feelings and physiological reactions elicited by a trauma reminder
Dialectical Behavior Therapy (DBT)	Treating borderline personality disorder, a syndrome often associated with PTSD and complex PTSD

In general, cognitive behavioral therapy is the most proven treatment for PTSD to date, although differences exist among various CBT approaches (as shown below). CBT treatments involve carefully scripted treatment manuals and usually require nine to 16 sessions. See individual approaches for specific efficacy studies to date.[30]

Prolonged Exposure (PE) Therapy

PE was developed to separate the traumatic memory from the conditioned emotional response so that the memory no longer dominates thoughts, feelings, and behavior. This approach uses both *imaginal* and *in-vivo exposure*.[30, 61-64]

Clinicians ask patients receiving imaginal exposure to narrate the traumatic event. If numerous traumatic episodes exist (as with survivors of recurrent child abuse, domestic violence, war trauma, or torture), the clinician asks patients to construct narratives about the worst events they clearly remember. The clinician prompts patients to close their eyes and visualize (imagine) what happened while repeating the narrative several times during a single session. Initially, patients will experience great anxiety as they begin to imagine themselves back in the traumatic situation. They are asked to rate the level of subjective distress every 10 minutes on a 10–100 *Subjective Units of Distress Scale* (SUDS), where 10 is no distress and 100 is the most fear/helplessness/horror they have ever experienced. Distress levels are usually in the 70–90 range during initial imaginal exposure sessions. However, through repeated exposure to the traumatic memory, patients experience a

imaginal exposure — systematically assisting trauma survivors to confront distressing trauma memories though the use of mental imagery

in-vivo exposure — patients practice techniques learned in therapy in the environment that represents their most-feared situation

Subjective Units of Distress Scale — a scale ranging from 10–100 with 10 being the least anxiety provoking and 100 being the most anxiety provoking. The SUDS scoring system allows the patient to express exactly how upsetting or distressing certain stimuli are in comparison to other anxiety experiences

An interesting variant of PE is virtual reality exposure therapy, which uses a computer-generated visual, auditory, and kinesthetic model of the patient's own traumatic experience.[65]

progressive reduction in distress levels so that they may fall to the 10–20 range by the end of a single session and remain at negligible levels by the end of an 8- to 10-session exposure therapy treatment. Following successful exposure treatment, patients can confront traumatic memories without having the recollections trigger intrusive and/or hyperarousal PTSD symptoms.

When ready, patients are encouraged, as part of a homework assignment, to confront situations associated with their traumatic experiences in the context of in vivo exposure.[30, 64]

PE may not be for everyone; some patients are either not ready or not willing to confront traumatic reminders and the intense anxiety provoked by this technique.

PE, with or without cognitive therapy, has been tested with survivors of a greater variety of traumatic events, including sexual assault, war-zone exposure, or childhood sexual abuse, than other treatments.

Efficacy — PE has consistently proven superior to supportive counseling or untreated patients monitored while on a "waiting list" for therapy. It is equal in efficacy to other forms of CBT treatment; results have shown 60 to 70 percent improvement in all three PTSD symptom clusters with improvements generally maintained six and 12 months later.[61, 65-69]

Cognitive Therapy

Cognitive therapy addresses thoughts and beliefs generated by the traumatic event rather than conditioned emotional responses addressed by exposure therapy.[61, 64–67, 70, 71] This approach focuses on how individuals with PTSD have interpreted the traumatic event with respect to their appraisals about the world and themselves. For example, those who have been overwhelmed by a catastrophic stressor typically perceive the world as dangerous and themselves as incompetent. As a result, PTSD patients see themselves as perennial victims powerless to cope with life and take charge of their personal destiny. Such a belief system then becomes a hard-wired, self-fulfilling prophecy.

Clinicians often combine cognitive therapy with exposure therapy to work on both conditioned emotional responses and automatic dysfunctional thoughts. One somewhat different approach for combining cognitive and exposure therapy is cognitive processing therapy (CPT).

Case Study Notes

Mary T.'s persistent inability to overcome her PTSD symptoms and resume her life as before has destroyed her confidence in herself. She has come to think of herself as a failure, someone unable to cope with even minor stressors. Because of this pervasive sense of personal inadequacy, she is easily overwhelmed and unable to perform routine tasks. It is a vicious circle since the more she fails to perform, the more she feels inadequate, and the more she finds the world overwhelming.

In cognitive therapy, the first step is to identify automatic thoughts (such as Mary's thoughts about herself) and to understand that, although originally developed from the trauma, these thoughts currently hinder adaptive functioning. Second, the therapy focuses on correcting erroneous thoughts with more accurate information, replacing automatic, dysfunctional thoughts with more realistic and adaptive ones. Successful cognitive therapy creates an accurate appraisal of:

> ► Situations perceived as either safe or dangerous rather than automatically perceiving all external events as dangerous

Case Study Notes

Mary needs to learn that there is nothing inherently dangerous about trucks or about driving a car. She needs to separate the specific tragic circumstances of her personal trauma from the trauma-related generalizations that currently make her afraid to travel on the highway.

> ► One's own strengths and weaknesses in different situations rather than an automatic belief that one is personally incompetent and unable to cope with life's challenges

Case Study Notes

Mary needs to understand that what happened during the accident was not due to a failure on her part and to learn that her current immobility is due to PTSD and not due to her own personal inadequacies.

Efficacy — Several studies comparing cognitive therapy with PE (alone and in combination) found equal effectiveness, producing 60 to 70 percent improvement in PTSD symptoms. Additionally, these individual or combined approaches outperformed relaxation therapy.[61, 65, 67, 72, 73]

Cognitive Processing Therapy (CPT)

CPT also uses written narratives to address both the emotional and cognitive consequences of trauma exposure so that patients can access and process the natural emotions that have been distorted and obscured by their personal interpretations of the traumatic event.[61, 74, 75]

According to CPT theory, negative belief systems that a person generates following a trauma (e.g., "I am powerless," "I am inadequate," "The world is a dangerous place") make it impossible to process normal emotional reactions to the catastrophic event (e.g., sadness and fear). This happens because the trauma survivor is preoccupied with inappropriate and intolerable emotions (e.g., guilt and shame) evolving from erroneous beliefs and interpretations about the traumatic experience. By confronting distorted traumatic memories, patients challenge/modify these erroneous beliefs, thereby dissipating inappropriate emotions.

CPT is similar to exposure therapy except the narratives are written by patients rather than elicited by the clinician. The written format gives the CPT patient more control over the pace and intensity of disclosure than is the case in exposure treatment.

> **Case Study Notes**
>
> Mary T.'s inappropriate feelings of guilt about the accident and shame about her current feelings of inadequacy have dominated her feelings about the traumatic event. They have prevented her from normal grieving about the loss of her husband, her marriage, her future, and the person she was before the accident. Psychological recovery depends upon moving beyond trauma-engendered cognitive distortions and inappropriate emotions so that she can freely process normal emotions (e.g., sadness and fear) that have been inaccessible up to this point.

Efficacy — In studies conducted with patients having rape-related PTSD, CPT performed as well as PE initially and six and 12 months after. All patients had significant reduction in all three PTSD symptom clusters, and none continued to meet PTSD diagnostic criteria at the six-month follow up. A recent, very large study comparing both approaches demonstrated equal effectiveness.[61, 68, 74]

Stress Inoculation Training (SIT)

Originally adapted for treating rape victims, SIT provides PTSD patients with a repertoire of tools and skills they can utilize to control anxiety elicited either by trauma-related stimuli or during threatening situations.[76, 77] It combines a variety of anxiety management techniques including relaxation and biofeedback training (see page 41). In addition, SIT utilizes:[61]

SIT aims to reduce avoidance behavior through anxiety reduction and foster a sense of personal competence.

- ▶ **Social skills training** — Clinicians help patients increase specific interpersonal skills necessary for positive relationships.

- ▶ **Role-playing** — Clinicians and patients practice responses to specific situations.

- ▶ **Distraction techniques** — Clinicians teach patients to yell "stop" to themselves each time certain thoughts start.

Efficacy — Four studies on women with rape-related PTSD or male or female motor vehicle accident survivors tested SIT alone or in combination with PE. In all cases, results from SIT were equal to those from PE, producing a 60 to 70 percent reduction in PTSD symptom severity. Three-month follow-up assessments showed substantial improvement in one study and improvement slightly better with PE than SIT in another study.[69, 74, 78, 79]

Interapy[80]

Given avoidant behavior that characterizes PTSD, growing Internet access worldwide, and the shortage of skilled CBT clinicians, interapy has much to recommend it for addressing the spectrum of post-traumatic distress, from acute stress reactions to PTSD.

Interapy is an Internet approach that modifies standard CBT (especially CPT) components (e.g., psychoeducation, exposure, and cognitive therapies) for this unique medium. Thus far, it has only been tested in the Netherlands. Interapy involves 10 sessions (twice a week for five weeks), where patients submit essays (approximately 450 words) to a Web site and receive clinician feedback. Major components are exposure/"self confrontation" and cognitive reappraisal much along the lines of CPT.

Efficacy — There have been two controlled trials of interapy, one with students and one with 184 Dutch participants, who reported mild-to-severe, post-traumatic symptoms. Neither study included formal PTSD diagnostic assessment; however, researchers observed a 50 percent or greater improvement in PTSD, depression, and other symptoms.[80, 81] More rigorous testing is needed for this exciting treatment option.

Imagery Rehearsal Therapy (IRT)[82]

IRT was developed to decrease the traumatic nightmares central to PTSD, reduce insomnia, and decrease PTSD symptom severity. IRT treatment consists of three weekly sessions in which patients learn cognitive-behavioral techniques for replacing unpleasant images with pleasant ones. Then they focus on a single, intolerable nightmare and are instructed to "change the nightmare" in any way they wish. Finally, they rehearse this new dream five to 20 minutes every day.

Efficacy — Four randomized **IRT** trials with crime victims, sexually abused adolescent girls and women, and Vietnam veterans have reported 50 to 60 percent reduction in nightmare frequency and overall PTSD symptom severity.[82–84] Further testing is needed, but IRT appears to be a promising, unique approach for PTSD patients experiencing nightmares.

Biofeedback and Relaxation Training[61]

Biofeedback is a process to reduce tension and anxiety in which the patient is given information about her/his own physiological processes. For example, the patient is given continuous feedback about heart rate, or muscle tension. S/he learns to consciously control these processes. Success is demonstrated by reductions in heart rate, muscle tension, or other physiological processes. Relaxation training is a treatment in which patients learn to relax their musculature through breathing and meditation-like tensing and untensing exercises, often assisted by audio tapes. Learning to induce muscle relaxation at will is used as a technique to control anxiety, when it occurs.

Efficacy — **Biofeedback and relaxation training** are ineffective stand-alone treatments but function as anxiety management techniques used with other CBT approaches, such as stress inoculation training (SIT) (reviewed on page 40).[61]

*See page 23 for more info on
establishing trust and safety.*

*For a specific model for
integrating DBT with prolonged
exposure for PTSD, refer to
one recently proposed by
C. B. Becker and C. Zayfert.*[87]

Dialectical Behavior Therapy (DBT)[27, 37]

DBT is a comprehensive CBT approach designed specifically for patients with *borderline personality disorder* and other difficult-to-treat patients too unstable to adhere to other treatments. Since DBT candidates often have significant trauma histories and often meet diagnostic criteria for PTSD or complex PTSD, this option may be appropriate for the initial stabilization (e.g., establishing trust and safety) phase of PTSD treatment.

DBT patients acquire skills to reduce chronic impulsive behavior marked by chaotic life problems, suicidal behavior, emotional lability, substance abuse, binge eating, and frequent hospitalizations. DBT is characterized by a balanced and flexible approach to therapy based on a strong patient-clinician relationship through which problem behaviors are explicitly addressed.

Efficacy — Although a number of reports describe moderate improvement for complex PTSD patients receiving DBT for suicidal, self-mutilating, impulsive, self-damaging, and binge-eating behaviors, no specific reports exist on DBT as a first-line or adjunctive treatment.[27, 37, 85, 86]

Eye Movement Desensitization and Reprocessing (EMDR)

Proponents of EMDR believe that *saccadic eye movements* reprogram brain function so that the emotional impact of a trauma can be finally and completely resolved.[88, 89] When conducting EMDR, the clinician instructs the patient to imagine a painful, traumatic memory and an associated negative cognition (e.g., guilt, shame). Then, the patient is asked to articulate an incompatible positive cognition (e.g., personal worth, self efficacy, trustworthiness). The clinician then has the patient contemplate the traumatic memory while visually focusing on the rapid movement of the clinicians' fingers. After each set of 10–12 eye movements, the clinician asks the patient to rate the strength of both the distressing memory and his/her belief in the positive cognition.

Despite the name of this therapy, research evidence suggests that eye movements do not appear necessary for EMDR to work.[90, 91] In published studies comparing conventional EMDR to EMDR minus eye movements, patients who received EMDR minus eye movements did just as well as those who received conventional EMDR. Therefore, it is difficult to substantiate that eye movements form the crucial ingredient in EMDR and even more difficult to defend the hypothesis that EMDR reprograms the brain's processing of traumatic memories.

Because empirical evidence suggests that EMDR is effective in treating PTSD (despite the apparent unimportance of eye movements), more research is needed to understand the actual mechanism by which EMDR works. Some theorists believe that EMDR is actually a variant of CBT. In practice, it does have some unique components that may account for its appeal among clinicians as well as its therapeutic efficacy. Most notable is the practice of having patients select the traumatic material, which they process in their own ways and at their own paces — in contrast to other approaches.[92]

Efficacy — EMDR appears to be more effective than no treatment among patients assigned to a wait list. It is also superior to psychodynamic, relaxation, or supportive therapies.

Published results indicate that following treatment, 50 to 77 percent of those receiving EMDR no longer met criteria for the PTSD diagnosis in comparison to 20 to 50 percent receiving supportive therapy or treatment-as-usual.[91, 93, 94]

Results are mixed regarding the relative efficacy of EMDR and CBT. Although head-to-head comparisons of the two treatments suggest that CBT produces better and longer-lasting outcomes, other studies suggest that both are comparable.[91, 95, 96] However, four meta-analyses have concluded that both are generally equally effective.[96–99]

Several studies have shown that, in comparison with wait list patients (who show little improvement), approximately two-thirds of those receiving EMDR no longer met PTSD diagnostic criteria.[91, 93, 94]

EMDR proponents argue that their treatment is not only as effective as CBT, but that it is shorter and better tolerated by patients.

Psychodynamic Psychotherapy

For over 100 years, clinicians have used psychodynamic psychotherapy to treat post-traumatic disorders. Psychodynamic theory focuses on *psychic balance*, which sometimes requires the patient to force intolerable thoughts and feelings out of conscious awareness through the process called *repression*. However, these now-unconscious traumatic memories are still powerful enough to become expressed as symptoms, such as PTSD's intrusion, avoidant/numbing, and hyperarousal symptoms.[100]

Psychodynamic treatment seeks to understand the context of the traumatic memories and the defensive processes through which the unconscious transforms repressed memories into the maladaptive symptoms that initially drive treatment. According to psychoanalytic theory, simply focusing on symptom reduction can achieve little as long as repressed memories remain.[100]

A new, healthier balance must be achieved by confronting unconscious processes that have repressed the memories and produced maladaptive compromises (e.g., symptoms). As these feelings, behaviors, and memories are explored, patients gain insight or understanding of how their repressed memories (along with associated thoughts and feelings) have been transformed into their current symptoms. This awareness ideally enables patients to exercise more control over the repression defense and thereby achieve symptom reduction.

psychic balance — a dynamic equilibrium state between those thoughts, feelings, memories, and urges the conscious can tolerate and those it cannot

repression — a hypothetical, unconscious process by which unacceptable (often trauma-related) thoughts and feelings are kept out of conscious awareness

Psychodynamic treatments vary from 10–20 sessions to open-ended treatment lasting many years. Longer psychodynamic treatments seek to create a fundamental change in psychic balance while briefer forms (12–15 sessions) seek to foster improved self-understanding and ego-strength.

Brief Psychodynamic Psychotherapy (BPP), conducted within 12–15 sessions, focuses on the traumatic event itself. Through the retelling of the trauma story to a calm, empathetic, compassionate, and non-judgmental clinician, the patient achieves a greater sense of *self-cohesion*, develops more adaptive defenses and coping strategies, and successfully modulates intense emotions that emerge during therapy.[104] While working through the traumatic memories, the clinician also addresses the linkage between post-traumatic distress and current life stress. Patients learn to identify current life situations and environmental triggers that set off traumatic memories and exacerbate PTSD symptoms.

self-cohesion — knowledge and integration of previously unconscious motivations

In some ways, BPP has similar goals to PE/CBT yet different conceptual underpinnings and therapeutic techniques.

Efficacy — Because psychodynamic treatment focuses primarily on psychic processes rather than psychiatric symptoms, there exists only one randomized clinical trial on treatment efficacy for reducing PTSD symptoms.

Much more research is needed to demonstrate psychodynamic treatment efficacy for PTSD.

This study involved the use of BPP for 18 sessions and compared results with hypnotherapy and CBT (systematic desensitization). BPP effectively reduced PTSD intrusion and avoidance symptoms by approximately 40 percent. This improvement was:[105]

- ▶ Sustained for three months
- ▶ Comparable to results from the other two treatments
- ▶ Significantly greater than a wait list group that received no treatment

Group Therapies

Group therapies utilize a psychodynamic focus, CBT focus, or supportive techniques (each with a different focus) and can be combined with the other therapies.[106] In all cases, trauma survivors learn about PTSD and help each other with the aid of a professional clinician.

Group therapy is effective and popular for those who have all survived the same type of trauma (e.g., war, rape, torture, terrorist bombing, etc.). As members share experiences, they become connected to one another by recognizing their common human fears, frailties, guilt, shame, and demoralization. Through clinician guidance, validation and normalization of these thoughts, feelings, and behaviors progresses to acquisition of more adaptive coping strategies, symptom reduction, and/or derivation of meaning from the traumatic experience.

Psychodynamic Focus Group Therapy

Group members help one another understand how their assumptions about themselves (e.g., weak, shameful, guilty, undeserving) have been shaped and distorted by their traumatic experiences. By revisiting this material in the safety of the group, they are empowered to confront the traumatic memories to gain new insight about these memories and themselves, and integrate such knowledge into their lives. Personal growth results from improved ego strength and self-understanding. While symptom reduction is not the major treatment goal, theorists expect resolution of trauma-related disruptions to normal psychic processes will promote PTSD amelioration.[107]

Efficacy — There is very little empirical research with psychodynamic focus group treatment for PTSD, and the few findings that have been reported are equivocal. In the one study of psychodynamic group treatment with childhood sexual abuse survivors, PTSD symptom severity was reduced by 18 percent.[108]

Cognitive Behavioral Focus Group Therapy

These groups embody the concepts and approaches described earlier for individual cognitive behavioral therapy (see pages 36–42).[75, 109] One specific group approach uses PE and CBT, where the clinician guides one group member at a time through a typical exposure session followed by cognitive restructuring.[110] During the exposure session, the other members are vicariously exposed to their own traumatic memories through observing someone else's treatment.

Group members do more for each other than provide social support. They validate one another's post-traumatic reactions, share their struggles to cope with PTSD-related problems, and provide honest criticism of fellow members' maladaptive coping behavior based on accurate empathy and their own experiences. Since group time is limited, group members must carry out homework assignments in which they focus or expose themselves to traumatic material. This homework is done through writing exercises or by repeatedly listening to an audio tape previously recorded during a group session in which they underwent exposure to their own traumatic material.

Efficacy — There is a great deal of empirical support for cognitive behavioral focus group treatment. In three studies of CBT group treatments (including CPT, assertiveness training, and SIT) on women traumatized by childhood or adult sexual abuse, PTSD symptoms were reduced 30 to 60 percent with reductions in all PTSD symptom clusters measured. Improvement was sustained for six months in all studies.[74, 77, 106] One CBT group treatment for combat veterans showed a 20 percent reduction in PTSD symptom severity.[111]

> *During the retelling of the trauma story, emotion is mobilized; as a result, the patient hopefully experiences a profound catharsis or "abreaction." Achieving catharsis is an important mediator of recovery in this treatment approach.*

> *The ultimate goal for both psychodynamic and cognitive-behavioral group therapy is for group members to gain "authority" over traumatic material so that it no longer becomes a dominant factor in their lives.[106]*

> *Other group approaches employing CBT have been utilized. Most notably CBT (see pages 36–37) and SIT (see page 40).[74, 77]*

> *There is also a report of group EMDR treatment for Vietnam War veterans.[107]*

Supportive Group Therapy

Supportive Group Therapy provides psychoeducation and focuses on members' current life issues.[106, 107] The goal of treatment is not to revisit, reframe, or master traumatic material, but to discuss here-and-now issues. Traumatic consequences, as expressed by PTSD symptoms, are only relevant if they affect present-day functioning. To improve emotional and interpersonal comfort and overall functioning, group members are encouraged to develop better interpersonal and coping skills, problem-solving skills, and more adaptive responses to predictable challenges.

Efficacy — In a recent, large randomized trial in which 360 Vietnam combat veterans with PTSD were randomized to 30 weekly sessions of either CBT or supportive therapy, results were similar for both groups. Thirty-eight percent of the veterans improved, 43 percent were unchanged, and 18 percent had worse symptoms after treatment.[112]

Additionally, one controlled trial of supportive group therapy for female sexual assault survivors showed a 19 to 30 percent reduction in intrusion and avoidance symptoms that was maintained for six months.[74]

Untested Treatments

A number of treatments, found effective for other psychiatric disorders, have not been tested systematically with PTSD patients. However, those often utilized in PTSD treatment despite lack of efficacy evidence are:

- ► **Couples/Family Therapy** — This treatment focuses on how relationships can either be disrupted by a family member's PTSD (systemic treatment) or foster a better healing environment for the PTSD patient (supportive treatment).[113–119]

- ► **Hypnosis** — Although no longer considered a PTSD treatment, hypnosis has demonstrated equal efficacy with both CBT (systematic desensitization) and psychodynamic psychotherapy in the single randomized trial.[105] It is now utilized primarily as an adjunctive procedure for confronting difficult traumatic memories, nightmares, or dissociative symptoms.[120]

- ► **Social Rehabilitative Therapies** — Effective for those with persistent mental illnesses (e.g., schizophrenia, severe affective disorders), these therapies are used with chronic, severe, and incapacitating PTSD (often indistinguishable from other persistent mental illness).[16, 121]

The seven psychosocial rehabilitation techniques recommended for severe and chronic PTSD are:[122]

1. Patient education services
2. Self-care/independent living skills techniques
3. Supported housing services
4. Family support
5. Social skills training
6. Supported employment techniques/ sheltered workshops
7. Case management

What Psychological Treatments are Available for Children and Adolescents with PTSD?

Treatments for children and adolescents are often age-appropriate interventions extrapolated from adult treatment methods. For children who develop PTSD, the impact of the trauma as well as the expression of symptoms may be significantly affected by the developmental stage at which the trauma occurred.[123] For example:

- **Abused infants and toddlers** may have impaired ability to form attachments with significant others.

- **Traumatized preschoolers**, who lack the conceptual and communication capacities of older individuals, may express nonverbal symptoms (e.g., aggression, withdrawal, or sleep problems).

- **Trauma in children** may result in restructured emotional expression, social isolation, problems with impulse control, self-injurious behaviors, dissociation, and development of *dissociative identity disorder* or borderline personality disorder.

- **Trauma during adolescence** may severely disrupt normal adult development by producing problems in separation from parents, personality evolution, symbolic thinking, and moral development.[124–128]

dissociative identity disorder — previously called multiple personality disorder, which is characterized by one's personality becoming so fragmented that pronounced changes in behavior and reactivity are noticed between different social situations or social roles

Treatment Efficacy for Children and Adolescents

A consistent body of evidence supports the efficacy of CBT treatment for children with PTSD.

There has been very little research on treatment for children with PTSD. However, the strongest findings, to date, indicate that the best results are achieved when the family is included in treatment, and that school-based treatments may offer the most efficient and effective approach for many children.[128–130]

Several experts have written thoughtful articles on developmentally sensitive treatment approaches for children with PTSD.[123] There is very little empirical evidence to guide us. Randomized trials of 10–18 sessions of CBT with children exposed to sexual trauma, natural disasters, and single-incident stressors, such as criminal assault or an automobile accident, have shown this approach superior to comparison treatments.[129–133] Among these, three studies on CBT group interventions in the school setting have shown impressive results:

1. In a study of nine- to ten-year-old survivors of the 1989 earthquake in Armenia, 20 to 40 percent experienced reduced PTSD symptoms compared to a non-treatment control group of children, whose symptoms worsened over the subsequent 18 months.[132]

2. An impressive, 18-week, school-based group CBT treatment was offered to children (grades four to nine), who had been exposed to a single-incident stressor (e.g., criminal assault, car accident, natural disaster — in contrast to protracted physical or sexual abuse). By the end of treatment, 57 percent no longer met PTSD diagnostic criteria; at the six-month follow-up, 86 percent no longer had PTSD.[133]

3. A school-based approach among Hawaiian children exposed to Hurricane Iniki successfully reduced PTSD intrusion and avoidance symptoms by 30 to 35 percent.[131]

Another school-based CBT approach successfully reduced depressive and anxiety symptoms among sexually abused preschool children, but PTSD symptoms were not monitored.[16]

It is important to include parents in treatments for children with PTSD. Many studies have shown that the parents' emotional reaction to the trauma and the amount of family support available to the child will have a significant impact on the child's symptoms.[134] The best predictor of a favorable outcome for children is if parents and other significant adults can cope with the trauma.[128] Therefore, psychoeducation and supportive family therapy described earlier (see pages 33–35 and page 46) are especially relevant to PTSD treatment for children.[130, 134]

play therapy — a technique for treating young children in which they reveal their problems on a fantasy level with dolls, clay, and other toys

Other approaches, such as *play therapy*, SIT, and psychoeducation, have primarily been the subject of speculation and uncontrolled clinical trials but have not been tested rigorously.

Key Concepts for Chapter Four:

1. Psychoeducation helps patients understand that their symptoms reflect a response to catastrophic stress shared by many as well as the nature of the disorder and its impact on their lives. It is especially useful as a societal and community intervention, using mass media, following terrorism or mass casualties due to a natural disaster.

2. Psychoeducational interventions help patients achieve normalization in their lives, remove self blame and doubt, correct misunderstandings about what's causing their symptoms, and enhance the clinician's credibility as someone who truly understands the patient's struggles.

3. Individual psychotherapy used to treat PTSD includes cognitive behavioral treatments (CBT), eye movement desensitization (EMDR), and psychodynamic psychotherapy. Of these, research suggests that CBT approaches are the most effective.

4. Prolonged exposure therapy (PE), which focuses on the details of the traumatic event itself, and cognitive therapy, which focuses on changing how the patient perceives the traumatic event, appear to be equally effective for improving PTSD symptoms (60–70 percent) when studied alone and in combination.

5. Despite mixed results for how EMDR impacts PTSD symptoms, empirical evidence suggests that it is effective in treating PTSD, perhaps as effective as CBT.

6. It is difficult to determine effectiveness of psycho-dynamic treatment due to its focus on psychic processes instead of psychiatric symptoms, which are far more measurable.

7. Group therapies are most effective for people who have survived the same type of trauma (e.g., veterans). These approaches use either psychodynamic, CBT, or supportive techniques and can be combined with other therapies.

8. Children and adolescents with PTSD face additional treatment challenges based on their development stage when the trauma occurred and the impact of that stage on how they were able to put what was happening into some overall context. Family and school involvement appear critical to treatment success.

Chapter Five:
Pharmacological Treatments for PTSD

This chapter answers the following:

▶ **How Does the Human Stress Response Occur?** — This section details the neurobiology involved in the "Fight, Fright, or Freeze" reaction as well as in the "General Adaptation Syndrome."

▶ **What Psychobiological Abnormalities Occur in Those with PTSD?** — This section covers abnormalities of the adrenergic, HPA, and serotonergic systems as well as those involved with neurotransmission.

▶ **How can Medications Best be Used to Treat PTSD?** — This section discusses specific drugs available for PTSD treatment and their efficacy as well as treatment strategies.

MEDICAL treatments for PTSD target abnormalities in the multiple biological systems involved with a person's response to stress. This section reviews:

1. Psychobiology of the body's general response to stress
2. Abnormalities in the human stress response associated with PTSD
3. Specific medication treatments that target these abnormalities
4. Corresponding efficacy research

How Does the Human Stress Response Occur?

Through evolution, humans have acquired a number of biological mechanisms for coping with the many different kinds of stresses normally encountered in the course of a lifetime. The *amygdala* plays a key role in coordinating the response to threat or stress. It mobilizes a number of cortical and subcortical brain mechanisms, initially through activation of corticotropin releasing factor (CRF). CRF also ignites two major components of the human stress response — the "Fight, Flight, or Freeze" reaction and the "General Adaptation Syndrome."

amygdala — principal nucleus in the brain for appraising emotional input and threatening stimuli and then mobilizing protective, defensive, or escape behavior

Fight, Flight, or Freeze Reaction

This reaction refers to the mobilization of brain and *sympathetic nervous system* (SNS) mechanisms in response to a threat.[135] During this reaction, the heart pumps more blood to the muscles, which enables them to perform defensive ("fight"), escape ("flight"), or hiding ("freeze") movements necessary for

sympathetic nervous system — part of the autonomic nervous system that regulates arousal functions such as heart rate and blood flow

51

survival. This reaction begins in the brain via a complex array of neurobiological mechanisms that have evolved to detect danger, experience fear, and to set off a sequence of adaptive, defensive, escape, and hiding responses.

neurotransmitters — chemical messengers that transmit signals from one nerve cell to another to elicit physiological responses

adrenergic response — neuronal activation mediated by either norepinephrine (noradrenaline) or epinephrine (adrenaline)

Several important brain and SNS chemicals (*neurotransmitters*) that relay signals from one neuron to the next mediate the fight, flight, or freeze response, called an *adrenergic response* because norepinephrine and epinephrine are also called noradrenaline and adrenaline. Adrenergic agents augment or attenuate such responses in the brain, heart, blood vessels, and elsewhere.

Although the fight, flight, or freeze response was described more than 50 years ago with regard to the SNS and muscle activity, we have only recently come to understand how the brain responds to threat. When faced with a dangerous or stressful situation, the amygdala releases CRF, which activates the neurons in the locus coeruleus — a small cluster of nerve cells that contains most of the brain's adrenergic neurons. Locus coeruleus neurons activate brain centers (such as the hypothalamus, hippocampus, and cerebral cortex) that mediate arousal, emotional reactivity, and memory as well as the SNS, which instigates the fight, flight, or freeze response. This same hormone (CRF) activates an additional response to stress — the general adaptation syndrome.

See page 56 for an explanation of how neurotransmitters function.

The General Adaptation Syndrome

The general adaptation syndrome is the second major system that responds to stress.[136] It is a hormonal rather than a neurotransmitter response and focuses on the *hypothalamic-pituitary-adrenocortical (HPA) axis.*

hypothalamic-pituitary-adrenocortical (HPA) axis — three anatomic structures that participate collectively in the hormonal response to stress: the hypothalamus (in the brain), the pituitary gland, and the outer layer (cortex) of the adrenal gland

cortisol — a hormone that increases energy by raising blood glucose levels, decreases immune processes, and causes other metabolic and neurobiological actions

The hypothalamus — a small, midline nucleus on the underside of the brain — releases CRF into the bloodstream, which carries it rapidly to the nearby pituitary gland, provoking the release of adrenocorticotropic hormone (ACTH). ACTH is then carried by the blood stream to the adrenal gland (perched atop the kidney), which releases *cortisol*. Cortisol has been called the "stress hormone" because blood cortisol levels are elevated during the normal human response to stress.

Many other neurobiological systems also participate in the human stress response, including the immunological system, the thyroid system, and other neurotransmitter and hormonal systems.[137, 138]

Medications that enhance serotonergic activity are classified as selective serotonin reuptake inhibitors (SSRIs), some of which have proven effective in PTSD treatment.

The neurotransmitter, serotonin, is intimately involved in both adrenergic and HPA activity. Primarily located in the brainstem raphe nuclei, which have abundant reciprocal interactions with the adrenergic and many other brain neurotransmitter HPA systems, serotonin can facilitate the human stress response. The diagram on page 53 depicts major brain areas involved in this response.

Figure 5.1   Human Stress Response

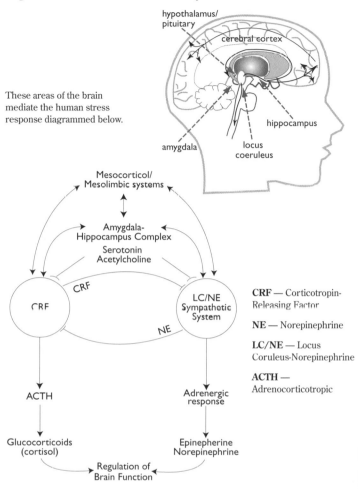

These areas of the brain mediate the human stress response diagrammed below.

CRF — Corticotropin-Releasing Factor

NE — Norepinephrine

LC/NE — Locus Coruleus-Norepinephrine

ACTH — Adrenocorticotropic

Diagram adapted from and reprinted with permission of Chrousos & Gold (1992).[137]

The following reviews abnormalities that result from trauma. On the horizon, research on medications that normalize the unique pathophysiology of PTSD appears promising. Such medications will most probably not be traditional antidepressants or anxiolytics, but pharmacological agents that act on CRF — a key component of the human stress response. CRF antagonists are important areas to develop to combat the entire human stress response. For example, neuropeptide Y enhancers that antagonize CRF actions might be another class of medications to test, as are other neuropeptides that affect these mechanisms.[15]

Since the systems affected by PTSD are key psychobiological mechanisms, advances in our basic understanding of human learning, memory, coping, and adaptation will accompany progress in this field.

What Psychobiological Abnormalities Occur in Those with PTSD?

The psychobiology of PTSD is complicated. Research indicates that other PTSD-related psychobiological abnormalities involve thyroid, opioid, immunological, and other neurotransmitter, neuropeptide, or neurohormonal systems. This chapter focuses only on the major systems altered in those with PTSD on which currently utilized pharmacological agents have the most influence. As we learn more about different brain mechanisms that PTSD affects, new medications will evolve to act on systems other than the adrenergic and serotonergic.

Research indicates that the adrenergic HPA and serotonergic systems as well as CRF function abnormally in people with PTSD.

Adrenergic System

For those with PTSD, it appears that the adrenergic (and SNS) system is much more active than in normal individuals. The most dramatic illustrations of this finding are experiments with *psychological* and *pharmacological* probes.

psychological probe — a visual or auditory stimulus reminiscent of a traumatic experience to which a person with PTSD is exposed

A typical psychological probe for a motor vehicle accident survivor with PTSD (such as Mary T. described in chapter two) may be the sound of a large truck or the squeal of brakes, the sight of a truck crashing into a car, or someone reciting details of a similar accident.[139, 140] Under such conditions, Mary T. would experience excessive SNS activation exhibited by a rise in blood pressure, a racing heart rate, and other physiological indications of heightened SNS physiological activity.

pharmacological probe — a drug that can activate psycho-biological mechanisms involved in the stress response

From the Patient's Perspective

I've been on the medication for three weeks now. I really didn't want to take it, but Dr. Owen convinced me that it might help me function better. It's really getting a lot easier to get behind the wheel of the car. I still don't like the trucks, but at least I can deal with them now. Therapy is really helpful. I can handle the memories a lot better and have begun to discover things that happened after the crash that I had completely forgotten. It's also easier to concentrate, and I can sit at the computer for a few hours. Dr. Owen wants me to consider easing back to work on a part-time basis. I don't think I'm ready, but I'll give it a try if she thinks I should.

Such physiological abnormalities can also cause abnormal elevations of blood or urinary norepinephrine as well as increased activations of the amygdala, locus coeruleus, and other brain centers. Mary T. may also experience abnormalities in the brain's normal blood flow; these include increased blood flow to the amygdala and reduced circulation to the pre-frontal cortex. Motor vehicle accident survivors who do not develop PTSD do not exhibit this heightened reactivity of adrenergic mechanisms in the SNS and brain.

A typical pharmacological probe is yohimbine, which causes excessive firing of adrenergic neurons.[138] Research with yohimbine has shown that the adrenergic system is abnormally sensitive in PTSD. Indeed, giving an intravenous dose of yohimbine to Mary T. might provoke a panic attack or even a flashback of the truck crashing into her car. Yohimbine does not produce such a response in people without PTSD. Yohimbine can even affect blood flow in the brain, thereby demonstrating the abnormal adrenergic sensitivity of those with PTSD.[141]

The prefrontal cortex is the part of the brain that exerts the major restraining influence on the amygdala.

HPA System

People with PTSD have shown a variety of HPA abnormalities, including elevated cerebrospinal CRF levels and abnormal serum and urinary cortisol levels (although study results are mixed).[142]

Although there is general agreement that those with PTSD have a significantly altered HPA system, there are a number of scientific controversies regarding the precise nature of HPA abnormalities. There is also evidence that people who develop PTSD have vulnerable HPA systems and that the traumatic event unmasked a biological abnormality that impairs their capacity to cope with catastrophic stress.[143]

Serotonergic System

Research with the serotonergic system in PTSD is at a much more preliminary stage than that with adrenergic or HPA mechanisms. It appears, however, that serotonin plays an important modulatory role on both systems, and is a key component of the human stress response.[138] Clinical studies show abnormalities in serotonergic mechanisms in PTSD patients.

synaptic cleft — the space between one neuron and the next that must be traversed by neurotransmitters

pre-synaptic neuron — the neuron that initiates neurotransmission by releasing the neurotransmitter into the synaptic cleft

post-synaptic neuron — the downstream neuron that is the target of neurotransmission

receptors — membrane-bound protein molecules with a highly specific shape that facilitate binding by neurotransmitters or medications

*An article entitled, "Pharma-cological Management of PTSD," (in **Primary Psychiatry**) offers a comprehensive review of PTSD pharmacology.*[144]

Neurotransmission

Medications used to treat PTSD modify neurotransmission in serotonergic and adrenergic neurons. Neurons communicate by releasing neurotransmitters into the *synaptic cleft*. The *pre-synaptic neuron* packages, releases, and delivers the neurotransmitter into the synapse, where it can diffuse across to the *post-synaptic neuron*.

Neurotransmitters attach to a specific post-synaptic *receptor*. The neurotransmitter forms a temporary binding complex with the receptor, analogous to a "lock-and-key" formation.

Binding of the neurotransmitter to the receptor results in a chemical change that leads to a biological response, such as a behavior, thought, or reaction.

After their pre-synaptic release, most neurotransmitters are subsequently re-absorbed by a specialized re-uptake site located on the pre-synaptic neuron. The re-uptake mechanism is selective for serotonin, or norepinephrine, respectively. Various medications affect different parts of the neurotransmitter system. These include:

- ▶ Selective serotonin reuptake inhibitors (SSRIs)
- ▶ Tricyclic antidepressants (TCAs)
- ▶ Venlafaxine
- ▶ Monoamine oxidase inhibitors (MAOIs)

Figure 5.2, below, illustrates what these medications block and the results. For more detailed information on these and other medications used to treat PTSD, review the following section.

Figure 5.2   Medication Impacts

Medications	What they Block	What's the Result
SSRIs	Pre-synaptic re-uptake site on serotonergic neurons	More serotonin available to bind post-synaptic receptors
TCAs Venlafaxine	Pre-synaptic re-uptake of both serotonin and norepinephrine	More neurotransmitters available to bind to post-synaptic receptors
MAOIs	Enzyme MAO, which destroys serotonin and norepinephrine	More neurotransmitters available to bind the post-synaptic, serotonergic, and adrenergic receptors

How can Medications Best be Used to Treat PTSD?

In view of the great success of cognitive-behavioral therapy (CBT), pharmacotherapy is only one of several treatment options for PTSD patients.[61] Medication may be a good choice when: [35]

> ▶ Patient acceptability of such an approach is high.

> ▶ Comorbid conditions are present that are responsive to pharmacotherapy (e.g., depression, panic disorder, social phobia, and obsessive-compulsive disorder).

> ▶ CBT treatment is unavailable.

Figure 5.3, on the following pages, summarizes the current clinical literature on pharmacological trials. It provides information on medication class, specific medication, therapeutic dose range, clinical indications, and contraindications. Of these medications, only two SSRIs are approved by the FDA for the treatment of PTSD (paroxetine and sertraline). SSRIs are considered the first-line treatment for PTSD because they:[144–146]

> ▶ Have broad-spectrum effects against all PTSD symptom clusters

> ▶ Are effective against many comorbid disorders

> ▶ Are effective against associated symptoms, such as impulsivity, aggression, and suicidal thoughts

Second-line medications include prazosin, MAOIs, TCAs, and venlafaxine. Evidence favoring the use of these agents is not as compelling as evidence for using SSRIs because of the lower numbers of participants tested.

Other medications included in the figure 5.3 include antiadrenergic agents and atypical antipsychotics. Laboratory research indicates a strong rationale for considering antiadrenergic agents; however, there will need to be more extensive testing to establish these agents' usefulness for PTSD patients. Atypical antipsychotics may effectively augment first- or second-line medication treatment; however, much more research is needed.

Chapter four provides detailed information on CBT treatment for those with PTSD.

Laboratory research indicates a strong rationale for considering antiadrenergic agents; however, there will need to be more extensive testing to establish these agents' usefulness for PTSD patients.

Atypical antipsychotics may effectively augment first- or second-line medication treatment; however, much more research is needed.

*Medications specifically **not** recommended for PTSD treatment include:*

> ▶ *Bupropion, mirtazapine — No systematic testing in clinical trials*

> ▶ *Carbamazepine, Valproate and Other Anticonvulsants — Only preliminary-stage research available*

> ▶ *Benzodiazepines — Appear ineffective against core PTSD symptoms*

> ▶ *Conventional Antipsychotics — Poor side-effect profile compared to other agents PLUS ineffective*

> ▶ *Nefazadone — Recently removed from U.S. market because of hepatotoxicity*

Figure 5.3   Medications for PTSD — Indications and Contraindications*

Class	Medication	Daily Dose Range (mg)	Indications	Contraindications
Selective Serotonin Reuptake inhibitors (SSRIs)	Paroxetine** Sertraline** Fluoxetine Citalopram Fluvoxamine	10–60 50–200 20–80 20–60 50–300	• Reduce B, C, and D symptoms • Produce clinical global improvement • Effective treatment for depression, panic disorder, social phobia, and obsessive compulsive disorder • Reduce associated symptoms (rage, aggression, impulsivity, suicidal thoughts)	• May produce insomnia, restlessness, nausea, decreased appetite, daytime sedation, nervousness, and anxiety • May produce sexual dysfunction, decreased libido, delayed orgasm, or anorgasmia • Clinically significant interactions with MAOIs • Significant interactions with hepatic enzymes produce other drug interactions • Concern about increased suicidal risk in children and adolescents
Other 2nd Generation Antidepressants	Trazadone Venlafaxine	150–600 75–100	• May reduce B, C, and D symptoms • Effective antidepressants • (Trazadone) Limited efficacy by itself but is synergistic with SSRIs and may reduce SSRI-induced insomnia • Preliminary multi-site trials indicate venlafaxine as effective as SSRIs	• (Trazadone) May be too sedating, rare priapism; however, may be useful as a bedtime medication for SSRI-induced insomnia.[142] • (Venlafaxine) May exacerbate hypertension
Monoamine Oxidase Inhibitors (MAOIs)	Phenelzine	15–90	• Reduces B symptoms • Produces global improvement • Effective agents for depression, panic, and social phobia	• Risk of hypertensive crisis requires a strict dietary regimen • Contraindicated in combination with most other antidepressants, CNS stimulants, and decongestants • Contraindicated in patients with alcohol/substance abuse/ dependency • May produce insomnia, hypotension, anticholinergic, and severe liver toxicity

B Symptoms: intrusive recollections
C Symptoms: avoidant/numbing
D Symptoms: hyperarousal

Figure 5.3 continued

Class	Medication	Daily Dose Range (mg)	Indications	Contraindications
Tricyclic Anti-depressants (TCAs)	Imipramine Amitriptyline Desipramine	150–300 150–300 100–300	• Reduce B symptoms • Produce global improvement • Effective antidepressant and antipanic agents • (Desipramine) Ineffective in one randomized clinical trial	• Anticholinergic side effects (dry mouth, rapid pulse, blurred vision, constipation) • May produce ventricular arrhythmias • May produce orthostatic hypotension, sedation, or arousal
Antiadrenergic Agents	Prazosin Propranolol Clonidine Guanfacine	6–10 40–160 0.2–0.6 1–3	• Reduces B and D symptoms • Produce global improvement • Prazosin shown to have marked efficacy for PTSD nightmares and insomnia	• May produce hypotension or brachycardia • Use cautiously with hypotensive patients; titrate prazosin starting at 1 mg at bedtime and monitor blood pressure • Propranolol may produce depressive symptoms, psychomotor slowing, or bronchospasm
Anticonvulsants	Carbamazepine Valproate Gabapentin Lamotrigine Topiramate	400–1600 750–1750 300–3600 50–400 200–400	• Effective on B, C, and D symptoms • Effective in bipolar affective disorder • Possibly effective in reducing aggressive behavior • Efficacy of gabapentin, lamotrigine, and topirimate not demonstrated in PTSD	• (Carbamazepine) Neurological symptoms, ataxia, drowsiness, low sodium, leukopenia, gastrointestinal problems, sedation, tremor, thrombocytopenia • (Valproate) Teratogenic and should not be used in pregnancy • (Gabapentin) Sedation and ataxia • (Lamotrigine) Stevens-Johnson syndrome, skin rash, fatigue • (Topiramate) Glaucoma, sedation, dizziness, ataxia
Atypical Antipsychotics	Risperidone Olanzapine Quetiapine	4–16 5–20 50–750	• Preliminary data: effective against PTSD symptom clusters and aggression • Potential role as augmentation treatment for partial responders to other agents	• Weight gain • (Olanzapine) Risk of type II diabetes

B Symptoms: intrusive recollections
C Symptoms: avoidant/numbing
D Symptoms: hyperarousal

*Modified from Friedman, 2003[144]
**FDA approval as indicated treatment for PTSD

The following discussion reviews medications considered first- and second-line agents in more detail.

Selective Serotonin Reuptake Inhibitors (SSRIs)

SSRIs have proven effective against other major DSM-IV psychiatric disorders that are frequently comorbid with PTSD, such as: depression, panic disorder, social phobia, and obsessive-compulsive disorder.

Two SSRIs, sertraline and paroxetine, have received FDA approval based on positive findings in large, 12-week, multi-site trials.[147–150] Improvement was found in 40 to 85 percent of respondents across trials. These agents offer many benefits, as shown in figure 5.3.

Sertraline and paroxetine are broad-spectrum medications, which ameliorate symptoms from all three PTSD symptom clusters (e.g., reexperiencing, avoidant/numbing, and hyperarousal).

More-recent findings indicate increased suicidal risk in children and adolescents taking SSRIs for depression.[154] However, comparable research for this age group is lacking among PTSD patients. However, given these findings, suicidal risk should be carefully monitored at all times. The FDA has recently issued a very strong warning concerning SSRI use for children and adolescents.[155]

SSRIs also appear to reduce clinically significant symptoms often associated with PTSD, such as suicidal, aggressive, and impulsive behavior. Finally, as with all SSRIs, sertraline and paroxetine have a side-effect profile that is relatively benign compared to other medications. A large, multi-site trial and smaller open trials with fluoxetine indicate that this SSRI is also a very effective PTSD medication.[151] Research with citalopram and fluvoxamine has also had favorable results.[146, 152]

Despite SSRIs' clinical advantages and relatively low side-effect profile (compared to other antidepressant agents such as MAOIs and TCAs), they are poorly tolerated by some patients. Sexual dysfunction, agitation, and insomnia produced by SSRIs, especially fluoxetine, may be especially disruptive to PTSD patients. In addition, clinicians should exercise caution when prescribing SSRIs to patients taking other medications (especially MAOIs) due to serious drug interactions and SSRI-induced disruption of normal drug metabolism in the liver. Finally, patients with gastrointestinal disorders, especially irritable bowel syndrome, sometimes experience problems when taking SSRIs because of increased intestinal motility.

Augmentation Strategies

▶ *Excessively aroused, hyper-reactive, or dissociating patients might benefit from augmentation with an antiadrenergic agent.*

▶ *Labile, impulsive, and/or aggressive patients might benefit from augmentation with an anticonvulsant.*

▶ *Fearful, hypervigilant, paranoid, and psychotic patients might benefit from an atypical antipsychotic.*

For patients who exhibit a partial response to SSRIs, one should consider continuation or **augmentation strategies**.[35] A recent trial with sertraline showed that approximately half of all patients failing to exhibit a successful clinical response after 12 weeks did respond when SSRI treatment continued for another 24 weeks.[153] Practically speaking, clinicians and patients usually will be reluctant to stick with an ineffective medication for 36 weeks, as in this experiment, making augmentation strategies more appealing.

Other Second-Generation Antidepressants

Venlafaxine, a powerful antidepressant that blocks pre-synaptic uptake of both serotonin and norepinephrine, appears to be very effective for PTSD, based on large, multi-site trials.[156]

Other second-generation antidepressants (e.g., bupropion and mirtazapine) are not recommended for PTSD treatment due to insufficient efficacy data. However, PTSD is often comorbid with major depression, and these medications are effective antidepressants with relatively benign side-effect profiles. Some clinicians automatically favor bupropion and mirtazapine over older agents despite the fact that both MAOIs and TCAs have proven effective for PTSD treatment, whereas bupropion and mirtazapine have not.

Monoamine Oxidase Inhibitors (MAOIs)

Comprehensive reviews of published findings on MAOI treatment indicate that MAOIs have produced moderate to good improvement in 82 percent of all patients, primarily due to reduction in reexperiencing symptoms, such as intrusive recollections, traumatic nightmares, and PTSD flashbacks.[157, 158] Insomnia also improved; however, avoidant/numbing or hyperarousal symptoms of PTSD did not.

Although tested infrequently, MAOIs have been very effective in most reported medication trials. Since they are also excellent antidepressants and antipanic agents, further research is definitely warranted.

MAOI use has traditionally been limited when there are legitimate concerns of patients ingesting alcohol or pharmacologically contraindicated illicit drugs or not adhering to necessary dietary restrictions — resulting in severe and abrupt elevation of blood pressure (a hypertensive medical emergency). Recent testing with a much safer MAOI, moclobemide, suggests that this may prove to be an effective drug for PTSD in the future.

A minimum of eight weeks of treatment with MAOIs or TCAs is necessary to achieve positive clinical results in veterans of military combat.

Tricyclic Antidepressants (TCAs)

In an analysis of all published findings on TCA treatment for PTSD, 45 percent of patients showed moderate to good global improvement following treatment, in contrast to MAOIs, which produced global improvement in 82 percent of patients who received them.[158] As with MAOIs, most improvement was due to reductions in reexperiencing rather than avoidant/numbing or arousal symptoms. Furthermore, TCAs' anticholinergic, hypotensive, sedating, and cardiac arrhythmic side effects are poorly tolerated by many PTSD patients.

Although TCAs are effective agents, side effects and failure to reduce avoidant/numbing symptoms have led to their replacement by SSRIs as first-line drugs in PTSD treatment.[145]

Antiadrenergic Agents

One of the earliest and most established findings in PTSD research is the excessive adrenergic reactivity among patients with the disorder.[141] Despite this robust, experimental finding and open trials dating back to 1984, antiadrenergic medications have been largely neglected until recently.[145]

The agents listed for this category in figure 5.3 (pages 58 through 59) are safe medications used for many years in treating cardiovascular disease, especially hypertension and cardiac arrhythmias. Although all agents listed achieve the result — reduced adrenergic activity — three different mechanisms of action account for this:

- ▶ **Prazosin** — A post-synaptic, alpha-1 receptor antagonist
- ▶ **Propranolol** — A post-synaptic, beta adrenergic antagonist
- ▶ **Clonidine and guanfacine** — Pre-synaptic, alpha-2 receptor agonists, which reduce the amount of norepinephrine released into the synaptic cleft

The best research on this class of agents (a well-controlled clinical trial) focuses on the alpha-1 antagonist, prazosin, which produced marked reduction in traumatic nightmares, improved sleep, and demonstrated global improvement among veterans with PTSD.[159] Tested in sexually/physically abused children with chronic PTSD, the beta antagonist, propranolol, significantly reduced (by 25–64 percent) reexperiencing and arousal symptoms.[160] Results with the alpha-2 receptor agonists, clonidine and guanfacine, are inconclusive despite laboratory evidence suggesting their potential effectiveness.[141] Clonidine has also been used successfully with Southeast Asian refugees with PTSD.[161]

Anticonvulsants

Much-needed research would include large-scale trials with these anticonvulsant/ antikindling agents (and other newly developed anticonvulsants) to clarify their usefulness in PTSD treatment.

Researchers hypothesize that following exposure to traumatic events, certain nuclei in the brain become "kindled" or "sensitized"; thereafter, they exhibit excessive responsivity to less-intense, trauma-related stimuli.[162] As with other medications, these results are preliminary at this time. In five studies, carbamazepine produced reductions in 50–75 percent reexperiencing and arousal symptoms, while in three studies, valproate produced reductions in 60–75 percent avoidant/numbing and 50–65 percent arousal (but not reexperiencing) symptoms.[163] These drugs have a clinically significant spectrum of neurological, *hematopoietic,* gastrointestinal, and *teratogenic* side effects that may restrict their usefulness for a number of patients. Since valproate's teratogenic effects occur early in the first trimester, it is best to discontinue this medication before pregnancy begins.

Given the theoretical importance of the kindling/sensitization model of PTSD and the complexity of clinical management with carbamazepine and valproate, current PTSD research has shifted to newer agents (such as gabapentin, lamotrigine, and topirimate).

Benzodiazepines

Clinicians often prescribe *benzodiazepines* for PTSD because of their proven efficacy as *anxiolytics.* This is unfortunate because studies with alprazolam and clonazepam indicate that these agents have **no proven efficacy against core PTSD symptoms**, whereas many more effective non-benzodiazepine agents are available, as reviewed previously.[145, 164] If prescribed, benzodiazepines typically improve sleep and reduce general anxiety, but have no salutary impact on the syndrome itself. Furthermore, there are **potential risks** of prescribing these agents because they may be problematic for patients with past or present alcohol/drug misuse. In addition, alprazolam may produce rebound anxiety, which is poorly tolerated by PTSD patients.

Antipsychotic Agents

Conventional antipsychotics are **not recommended for PTSD** patients, partly because more effective treatments are available and because *extrapyramidal* side effects make these agents a poor choice for PTSD treatment.[145]

Although there is very little data from clinical trials, preliminary studies suggest that **atypical antipsychotics** may be effective agents for PTSD global improvement, have selective action on B, C, or D symptoms, and reduce aggressive behavior.[145] Atypical agents, which have potent pharmacological actions but less-toxic, side-effect profiles, may have a unique niche as augmentation treatment for partial responders to SSRIs or other first- or second-line agents, especially for patients with intense hypervigilance/paranoia, agitation, dissociation, or brief psychotic reactions associated with their PTSD.[165]

---

hematopoietic — suppression of the bone marrow's capacity to produce red and white blood cells

teratogenic — producing fetal abnormalities during pregnancy

benzodiazepine family of drugs — a very effective and widely prescribed class of medications for anxiety that includes: diazepam, lorazepam, alprazolam, and clonazepam

anxiolytics — medications that relieve anxiety

extrapyramidal — uncontrollable involuntary motor movements or excessive rigidity

Many Vietnam veterans in the 1970s received conventional antipsychotic agents to ameliorate intense PTSD-related hyperarousal, hypervigilance, dissociative symptoms, aggressivity, and reexperiencing symptoms. However, we now understand that PTSD is pathophysiologically different from psychotic disorders.

Key Concepts for Chapter Five:

1. Humans respond to stress using biological coping mechanisms instigated by the amygdala, which promotes release of corticotropin releasing factor (CRF) and cortisol. These mechanisms involve the sympathetic and central nervous systems' adrenergic neurotransmitters and the hypothalamic-pituitary-adrenocortical axis as well as the immunological, thyroid, and other neurotransmitter and hormonal systems.

2. SSRIs represent the recommended, first-line approach to treating PTSD based on clinical evidence, with trazodone considered effective as augmentation therapy to SSRIs.

3. Second-line medications include venlafaxine, prazosin, TCAs, and MAOIs.

4. MAOIs have proven effective for treating PTSD; however, some symptoms appear unaffected and risk of a hypertensive reaction can be problematic.

5. Side effects associated with anticonvulsants and atypical antipsychotics cause these two medication classifications to be considered as third-line agents for treating PTSD.

6. Pharmacotherapy is the most reasonable approach to PTSD treatment when patients are strongly in favor of taking medications, when comorbid conditions will also be addressed by the medications, and when CBT treatment is unavailable.

7. Benzodiazepines and antipsychotic agents are not recommended for treating PTSD, partly because of side effects and partly due to there being more effective treatments available.

Chapter Six:
Strategies for Acute Stress Reactions and Acute Stress Disorder (ASD)

This chapter answers the following:

▶ **What are Normal Acute, Post-Traumatic Distress Reactions?** — This section defines the four types of normal reactions people have to traumatic events.

▶ **What is Acute Stress Disorder (ASD)?** — This section defines ASD and presents prevalence information.

▶ **What Challenges Exist for Diagnosing ASD?** — This section covers risk factors for PTSD, differentiating ASD from PTSD, DSM-IV diagnostic criteria, and assessing ASD in clinical interviews using assessment and diagnostic tools.

▶ **What Treatment Approaches Are Used for Traumatic Event Survivors?** — This section covers immediate interventions as well as psychological and pharmacological interventions.

IMMEDIATELY after a traumatic event, those exposed may experience severe and incapacitating psychological distress — avoid traumatic stimuli and have startle reactions, hypervigilance, or other symptoms associated with PTSD. However, these distressing symptoms appear to be within the normal, immediate human response to overwhelming events.

Most people exposed to traumatic events never develop PTSD, depression, alcoholism, or any other DSM-IV(TR) psychiatric disorder. A recent review of 160 studies on disaster victims suggests that two-thirds will not develop a clinically significant chronic psychiatric disorder.[166–168] Most reactions were transient with symptom dissipation within a month of the disaster for 42 percent of the victims, and within a year for an additional 23 percent. Only a substantial minority, 30 percent, experienced chronic symptoms lasting more than a year.

Consider the reactions of two, U.S. World Trade Center disaster survivors, Kevin W. and William G.

▶ **Kevin**, who was lucky enough to flee his office in the South Tower shortly after the North Tower was hit, was not injured physically but witnessed terrifying death and destruction all around him.

▶ **William** was led from the 64th floor of the South Tower by firefighters and experienced all that Kevin had plus breathing problems from the smoke.

Both were extremely distressed during the immediate post-traumatic aftermath and might characterize their feelings as in the first "From the Patient's Perspective" box on the next page.

From the Patients' Perspective

Kevin W. or William G. — Immediate Post-Trauma Aftermath

It's been two days now, and I'm a nervous wreck. I know I should be thankful that I got out alive, but I'm climbing the walls. I jump at the slightest noise. I'm glued to the TV, and every time the instant replay shows those planes hitting the Twin Towers, I go into a panic, start to sweat, can't calm down, can't stop thinking about all those who didn't make it, and can't sleep because of the nightmares, can't stop smelling the awful smoke, and can't stop hearing the cries for help from those trapped on the upper floors.

However, what they report two weeks later (below) reflects symptoms that may differentiate an acute stress reaction (ASR) from an acute stress disorder (ASD).

From the Patients' Perspective

Kevin W. and William G. — Two Weeks Later

Kevin W.: Acute Stress Reaction

It's been two weeks since the Twin Towers were attacked. In the beginning, I couldn't seem to get a grip. Sally said, for the first few days, I was screaming in my sleep and thrashing about in the bed. When awake, she said I seemed to be off somewhere else when she tried to get my attention or comfort me. Thankfully, I've moved way beyond that point and no longer have the nightmares, anxiety, or spacey feelings. Although I'll never forget what happened, things are returning to normal, and my life continues to progress beyond September 11th.

William G.: Acute Stress Disorder

It's been two weeks, and I'm still not myself. I jump at the slightest sound, can't focus on anything at work or at home, can't sleep, and can't stop thinking about how my panic got even worse when I couldn't breathe because of the thick smoke in the stairway as I frantically tried to get out of the building. And, my internal world seems completely different. It's like living in a dream world instead of real life. I'm not connected to my feelings. It almost seems like I'm outside, looking in. Watching someone who looks like me but really isn't.

Most people (like Kevin W.) exposed to a traumatic event who exhibit Acute Stress Reaction (ASR) will recover spontaneously within a few days. Only a minority will develop ASD (like William G.), or some other psychiatric problem. However, since the vast majority of people who survive a catastrophic stressor will be very distressed during the immediate post-disaster aftermath, it is usually impossible to distinguish those who are most likely to recover on their own from those at greatest risk to develop a chronic psychiatric disorder.

This chapter considers this challenge and reviews current thinking about the best approach for ameliorating normal distress and treating clinically significant problems.

What are Normal Acute, Post-Traumatic Distress Reactions?

According to the National Center for PTSD Web site, www. ncptsd.va.gov, normal acute, post-traumatic reactions that last several days or weeks often consist of the following:

- ▶ **Emotional reactions** — Shock, fear, grief, anger, resentment, guilt, shame, helplessness, hopelessness, and numbing
- ▶ **Cognitive reactions** — Confusion, disorientation, indecisiveness, difficulty concentrating, memory loss, self-blame, and unwanted memories
- ▶ **Physical reactions** — Tension, fatigue, edginess, insomnia, startle reactions, racing heart beat, nausea, loss of appetite, and change in sex drive
- ▶ **Interpersonal reactions** — Distrust, irritability, withdrawal, and isolation; feeling rejected or abandoned; being distant, judgmental, or being over-controlling

These reactions may vary from mild to severe. In some cases, there is evidence of more clinical symptoms, such as: intrusive recollections, marked avoidance, dissociation, psychic numbing, panic attacks, intense agitation, incapacitating anxiety, severe depression, and grief reactions (over the death or injury of loved ones as well as personal material losses).

At an early stage, the appropriate professional stance is that these are transient reactions from which normal recovery should be expected.

Within three to five days of the September 11, 2001 World Trade Center attacks, 90 percent of Americans surveyed nationally reported at least moderate distress while 44 percent of respondents reported one or more substantial symptoms of severe distress.[169] In contrast to the high prevalence of normal post-traumatic distress, a much smaller percentage of New Yorkers, 7.5 percent, developed PTSD within weeks of the World Trade Center attacks.[170]

What is Acute Stress Disorder (ASD)?

*In Stephen Crane's novel about the Civil War, **The Red Badge of Courage**, the protagonist, a new recruit to the Union Army, has a classic attack of an acute stress reaction during his first exposure to enemy gunfire, from which he shortly recovers.*

Most people exposed to a traumatic event will exhibit psychological distress; for some this distress will be a transient acute stress reaction that may be briefly incapacitating, at most. For others, this distress may signal the start of a severe, chronic, and potentially incapacitating psychiatric disorder. The public health problem lies in distinguishing vulnerable from resilient individuals during the immediate aftermath of a terrorist attack, mass casualty, or natural disaster. Long ago, military psychiatrists named these acute reactions "combat stress reaction" or "battle fatigue."

Although most recover from "battle fatigue," a significant minority of people will experience persistent reactions and go on to develop PTSD after a month passes. Until the DSM-IV, there was no recognized diagnosis that could be given to an individual suffering high-magnitude and clinically significant distress during the immediate aftermath of a traumatic event. Today, the DSM-IV(TR) provides specific criteria for diagnosing ASD (see figure 6.2 on page 71).

In the only published study on children, only 12 percent with ASD developed PTSD at follow-up.[171]

Studies conducted shortly after disasters and other traumatic events found ASD in seven to 33 percent of survivors. More importantly, the incidence of ASD rather successfully predicts the later development of PTSD — overall, 70 to 80 percent of people with ASD will develop PTSD. However, approximately 60 percent of those who develop PTSD do so without ever meeting diagnostic criteria for ASD.[172–175]

Early detection is important for treatment as different interventions may be indicated for people depending on their level of vulnerability vs. resilience.

What Challenges Exist for Diagnosing ASD?

Currently, the lack of empirical research into prognosis and risk factors makes differentiation extremely difficult.

Risk Factors for ASD

Although little research data on risk factors exists for ASD, they are probably similar to those related to PTSD (see chapter two, page 16). In one study, risk factors identified were female gender, stress severity, depression, and an avoidant coping style.[13]

In addition, ASD has only limited usefulness as a screening criterion for the general population since most people who develop PTSD fail to meet ASD criteria beforehand.[176] This is a concern for public mental health planners who, understandably, want to neither make normal and transient post-traumatic symptoms pathologic nor use scarce and expensive clinical resources for individuals who will recover spontaneously or with minimal assistance.

PTSD and ASD symptoms are similar in terms of reexperiencing and hyperarousal symptoms (which are identical), and ASD avoidant symptoms (which are the same as the first two avoidant/numbing symptoms for PTSD). Differences involve emphasis, number of symptoms in each category, and definition of functional impairment. Figure 6.1, below, provides an at-a-glance reference for these differences.

Although not sufficiently tested, prognostic indicators for detecting how chronic symptoms might be are functional impairment, elevated heart rate, and negative cognitions.[168, 176–178]

Figure 6.1   Differences between ASD and PTSD

Differences	ASD	PTSD
Emphasis	Dissociative Symptoms	Avoidant and Numbing Symptoms
Number of Dissociative Symptoms	3 (including 1 numbing and 1 amnesia symptom)	0
Number of Avoidant Symptoms	1	3 (avoidant and numbing)
Number of Anxiety/ Arousal Symptoms	1	2
Onset/Duration of Symptoms	2 days to 4 weeks	Over 4 weeks
Functional Impairment	Clinically significant distress and functional impairment; unable to obtain necessary assistance	Clinically significant distress and impairment socially, occupationally, and in other important areas of functioning

It is the inclusion and prominence of dissociative symptoms that sets ASD distinctly apart from PTSD.

Distinguishing ASD from PTSD

The major difference between ASD and PTSD is the greater emphasis placed on symptoms of *dissociation*, which is characterized by normal mental functions (e.g., memory, a sense of time, or a sense of one's body or personal identity as a coherent entity) being severely distorted. To meet ASD diagnostic criteria, an acutely traumatized individual must exhibit **three** dissociative symptoms (criterion B symptoms), while it is possible to diagnose PTSD with none. These dissociative symptoms include:

dissociation — an abnormal cognitive/emotional state in which one's perception of oneself, one's environment, or the relationship between oneself and one's environment is altered significantly

1. **Reduction in Awareness** (Criterion B$_2$) — An individual's perceptions, thoughts, and feelings are focused internally rather than on external surroundings, appearing to onlookers as the individual being "in a daze," "spaced-out," or in a world of his/her own.

derealization — an alteration in the perception or experience of the external world so that it seems strange or unreal (e.g., people may seem unfamiliar or mechanical)

depersonalization — an alteration in the perception or experience of the self so that one feels detached from, and as if one is an outside observer of, one's mental processes or body (e.g., feeling like one is in a dream)

2. *Derealization* (Criterion B₃) — Typical perceptions of the external environment are significantly altered. One's sense of time may be accelerated or slowed down. People or objects appear to have lost their substance. The world one has always known is dramatically changed, and one feels estranged or detached from the environment or has a sense that the environment is unreal. For example, one may feel that familiar, routine places seem unfamiliar.

3. *Depersonalization* (Criterion B₄) — It appears that one's self, rather than one's world (as in derealization), has changed. Depersonalization may manifest itself as a distorted perception of one's body, identity, or self as a coherent entity (e.g., having an out-of-body experience of looking down on one's body from above; or feeling that one's body is split into sections: one part might be numb, another warm, and another cold).

4. **Numbing** (Criterion B₁) — In ASD, PTSD numbing symptoms (C₅₋₆), detachment and psychic numbing, are considered one (of five) dissociative symptom clusters.

5. **Amnesia** (Criterion B₅) — Likewise, in ASD, PTSD amnesia (C₃) is considered a dissociative symptom.

In addition to dissociative symptoms, ASD must last a minimum of two days and a maximum of four weeks, whereas PTSD cannot be diagnosed until at least four weeks after the traumatic experience.

Understanding DSM-IV Diagnostic Criteria

See page 10 for complete diagnostic criteria of PTSD.

ASD is a diagnostic classification for people experiencing significant psychological distress within one month of a trauma. Figure 6.2, on the next page, presents the DSM-IV (TR) diagnostic criteria for PSTD.

Conducting a Clinical Interview for ASD

The caution, sensitivity, and patience a clinician uses in a PTSD diagnostic interview must also be evident to the patient during an ASD assessment. The major difference, of course, is that the PTSD patient has a chronic condition to which the patient has had an opportunity to adapt, whereas ASD patients have been acutely traumatized, finding themselves in an intense, novel, and extremely disturbing psychological state difficult to comprehend. Patients may feel they are out of control and/or like they're losing their minds, perhaps exhibiting severe anxiety, agitation, and apprehension. Therefore, when conducting an ASD assessment, the clinician must initially approach it as carefully and thoughtfully as any other urgent or emergent psychiatric evaluation.

Figure 6.2   DSM-IV (TR) Diagnostic Criteria for Acute Stress Disorder[5]

A. The person has been exposed to a traumatic event in which both of the following were present:

1. the person experienced, witnessed, or was confronted with an event or events that involved actual or threatened death or serious injury, or a threat to the physical integrity of self or others

2. the person's response involved intense fear, helplessness, or horror

B. Either while experiencing or after experiencing the distressing event, the individual has three (or more) of the following dissociative symptoms:

1. a subjective sense of numbing, detachment, or absence of emotional responsiveness

2. a reduction in awareness of his or her surroundings (e.g., "being in a daze")

3. derealization

4. depersonalization

5. dissociative amnesia (i.e., inability to recall an important aspect of the trauma)

C. The traumatic event is persistently reexperienced in at least one of the following ways: recurrent images, thoughts, dreams, illusions, flashback episodes, or a sense of reliving the experience; or distress on exposure to reminders of the traumatic event.

D. Marked avoidance of stimuli that arouse recollections of the trauma (e.g., thoughts, feelings, conversations, activities, places, people).

E. Marked symptoms of anxiety or increased arousal (e.g., difficulty sleeping, irritability, poor concentration, hypervigilance, exaggerated startle response, motor restlessness).

F. The disturbance causes clinically significant distress or impairment in social, occupational, or other important areas of functioning or impairs the individual's ability to pursue some necessary task, such as obtaining necessary assistance or mobilizing personal resources by telling family members about the traumatic experience.

G. The disturbance lasts for a minimum of 2 days and a maximum of 4 weeks and occurs within 4 weeks of the traumatic event.

H. The disturbance is not due to the direct physiological effects of a substance (e.g., a drug of abuse, a medication) or a general medical condition, is not better accounted for by Brief Psychotic Disorder, and is not merely an exacerbation of a preexisting Axis I or Axis II disorder.

Empirical justification for including these three dissociative symptoms for ASD is sparse. It relies mostly on clinical observations and on evidence showing that people who experience acute dissociative symptoms during a traumatic event are at a greater risk for later developing PTSD.

Reprinted with permission by the American Psychiatric Association: *Diagnostic and Statistical Manual of Mental Disorder, Fourth Edition Text Revision.* Washington DC: American Psychiatric Association, 2000.

Using ASD Assessment and Diagnostic Tools

Appendix C details the available assessment and diagnostic tools for ASD.

Appendix C lists assessment and diagnostic tools for ASD and their applicability to adult vs. child patients. As with PTSD assessment tools (see page 17 and appendices A and B), ASD tools are divided into diagnostic instruments and symptom severity scales. PTSD trauma exposure scales will also serve for ASD as long as the clinician conducts the assessment within one month of the traumatic experience.

Counseling the Patient with an Acute Stress Reaction

In a first session following a traumatic event, the patient may be so distressed that the clinician will be unsure as to whether or not the patient will develop ASD or PTSD. Barring definitive symptoms for either disorder, preliminary counseling may involve providing educational information about acute stress reactions and recommending further contact if symptoms increase. This education typically stresses that what the patient is experiencing:

- ► Affects almost everyone exposed to catastrophic stress
- ► Usually resolves within days or weeks
- ► Typically does not lead to any permanent psychological scars or psychiatric problems

Key recommendations for these patients include:

- ► Avoiding re-exposure to traumatic reminders (e.g., not watching traumatic images on TV)
- ► Spending as much time as possible with friends and family
- ► Being patient so that normal recovery can take place

What Treatment Approaches are Used for Traumatic Event Survivors?

There is growing consensus that the best mental health intervention during the immediate aftermath of a traumatic event is *psychological first aid*, which would include:[179]

psychological first aid — an approach designed to ameliorate immediate post-traumatic distress based on the expectation that every survivor, no matter how upset, will achieve normal recovery

- ► Provision of basic needs — safety, security, and survival (food and shelter)
- ► Orientation to disaster and recovery efforts
- ► Reduction of physiological arousal through self-calming and relaxation techniques, avoiding upsetting stimuli, and (occasionally) taking medication

> ▶ Mobilization of support for those most distressed through reunion with family/friends and provision of needed professional services

> ▶ Providing education about available resources and coping strategies

> ▶ Using effective risk communication techniques to provide accurate, necessary information to survivors in a calm, honest, and straightforward manner without increasing anxiety

Following exposure to a traumatic event, individuals should be encouraged to live their lives as normally as possible and avoid isolating themselves from family, friends, or community-based natural support systems (e.g., neighborhood, school, church, or workplace organizations).

In the event of a natural or man-made disaster, public health approaches in the vicinity of the terrorist attack or disaster site should have both educational and outreach components.[180] Such large-scale, community/societal interventions should be designed to promote resilience and foster recovery among the majority of the population, temporarily suffering from acute post-traumatic reactions. They also need to provide widely accessible information about clinically significant post-traumatic symptoms so that people can make accurate appraisals concerning the magnitude of their own distress as well as that of loved ones and friends. Such a proactive approach should also indicate what type of mental health services might be helpful and where they can be found.

Information available through print and broadcast media, Internet sites, and toll-free telephone hotlines rank among key vehicles for carrying out such a public health approach.

PROJECT LIBERTY

New York City's post-9/11 disaster mental health program, Project Liberty, illustrates effective media-public health partnerships that benefit the general public after a major catastrophe. A broad-scale, public media campaign such as this should have four objectives:[181]

1. Branding a disaster-response program to provide recognition of available services

2. Broadcasting the overall message that post-traumatic distress is a normal reaction

3. Promoting a sense of security for the community at large by announcing that mental health services are available to those in need

4. Identifying and legitimizing outreach staff conducting face-to-face and door-to-door outreach services

Two weeks following the attack, Project Liberty developed and aired a 30-second TV commercial directing people to available mental health services. Within two months, 25 percent of New Yorkers knew about Project Liberty, and 70 percent reported that they had learned about it through television.[170]

Project Liberty also used radio announcements, printed brochures, a toll-free phone number, and information on the Internet. In addition, the project's community-directed interventions were tailored specifically for school children, the elderly, the workplace, and for many distinct ethnic communities.[181]

Psychological Interventions Used for Treating Acute Distress

There are many major gaps in early interventions research. Most research has focused on two approaches: psychological debriefing and brief cognitive behavioral therapy. Evidence for the former has been largely negative, while findings with four-to-five sessions of CBT have been very encouraging.

Psychological Debriefing

Many people believe that the best approach for those who experience a catastrophic event is early detection and timely intervention. This intervention is called *psychological debriefing*.

Proponents of psychological debriefing assert that it can abort the onset of a serious mental disorder, can reduce severity and duration once it has taken hold, or can prevent ASD from progressing to a chronic and incapacitating state.

Psychological debriefing was derived from military psychiatry. There clinicians found that active duty personnel who had an incapacitating anxiety attack (e.g., "battle fatigue" or "combat stress reaction") had better outcomes if treated at a medical unit close to the war zone, such as a mobile army surgical hospital (MASH) unit.[182] Thought to produce rapid resolution of battle fatigue and prevent the later development of what is now called PTSD, military psychological debriefing (P.I.E.) included three main components:

1. **Proximity** — Providing intervention at a location as close to the active combat zone as possible
2. **Immediacy** — Intervening as soon as possible after the onset of battle fatigue
3. **Expectancy** — Providing education that the acute stress reaction is a normal human response to an overwhelming and abnormal event, including the expectation that the individual will quickly recover and return to military duties within a few days without immediate or long-term consequences from the acute stress reaction

Although the military P.I.E. approach has not been rigorously tested, its apparent success fostered the use of similar interventions for civilians who experienced natural disasters or man-made catastrophes.

Psychological debriefing is often conducted in two-hour sessions with 10–20 participants, typically following this process:[183, 184]

▶ The group shares facts about the traumatic event.
▶ The group collectively reviews personal thoughts, impressions, and emotional reactions.

---

psychological debriefing — an intervention conducted by trained professionals shortly after a catastrophe, allowing victims to talk about their experience and receive information on "normal" types of reactions to such an event

The best known form of psychological debriefing is Critical Incident Stress Debriefing (CISD).[183] However, its many modifications and variations have led to use of the more general term, psychological debriefing.

▶ The facilitator informs participants that it is quite natural for some people to have disturbing symptoms shortly after a traumatic event.

Subsequently, group members are encouraged to speak about any such symptoms they may have experienced, then the group focuses on effective internal coping mechanisms and external (social) support.

▶ The facilitator distributes psychoeducational materials describing the normal human response to catastrophic stress and debriefs the group, generating a positive expectancy that disturbing, post-traumatic stress symptoms will probably subside within weeks.

▶ Group members receive lists of available mental health practitioners to contact if their symptoms do not subside.

According to proponents of psychological debriefing, this sharing of such intense personal information gives participants a chance to ventilate powerful feelings and learn that others have had similar reactions.

Psychological Debriefing Effectiveness in Preventing Later PTSD

Despite its popularity and history, research suggests that psychological debriefing recipients either receive no benefit or actually experience a worsening of their symptoms.[185, 186]

Eleven, rigorous, randomized clinical trials (RCTs) on psychological debriefing have been conducted thus far.[186, 186] In all cases, the intervention tested consisted of a single session of individual debriefing, administered within the first month after the traumatic event. In no case did debriefing prevent the later development of PTSD. In some cases, it appeared to delay recovery since comparison subjects who did not receive debriefing were less symptomatic at follow-up.[187, 188]

In spite of research to the contrary, most disaster survivors and clinicians who treat them feel that they benefited from the intervention. This is because most disaster survivors do not develop PTSD, whether or not they receive psychological debriefing.

Much more research must be done, especially since there are currently no published RCTs of group debriefings with groups of professional (military, firefighters, emergency medical) personnel in whom group cohesion and mutual support was established prior to the traumatic event.

Four theoretical reasons for the consistent failure (and possibly counterproductive) effect of debriefing on recovery are:

1. Forcing premature exposure to traumatic memories may actually interfere with a natural recovery process that allows the traumatic material to be consolidated and then to fade from conscious awareness.[178, 185, 189]

2. Debriefing during the immediate post-traumatic aftermath may actively interfere with habituation and cognitive changes that are essential for normal recovery.[178, 191]

3. An early focus on acute post-traumatic symptoms may foster negative cognitions about oneself (e.g., "Most people feel better by now so there must be something

Avoidance may be an important adaptive strategy in the very early stages of normal recovery from traumatic events and should not be disrupted by early interventions such as debriefing.[190]

wrong with me."). Negative cognitions predict the later development of PTSD.[192, 193]

4. Excessive post-traumatic adrenergic activity predicts PTSD because it facilitates the encoding of traumatic memories.[177, 194] Debriefing may activate such mechanisms thereby facilitating the encoding of intrusive memories that increase the risk for PTSD.[195]

Cognitive Behavioral Therapy

See pages 36–42 for a detailed description of CBT.

In contrast to negative findings with debriefing, at least five RCTs with CBT have had very promising results. These brief CBT interventions are usually not initiated until at least 14 days after acute traumatization; much later than the standard 72-hour, post-traumatic window in which debriefing is generally offered.

Brief CBT protocols of four or five sessions that include both exposure therapy and cognitive restructuring have been shown to ameliorate ASD or acute post-traumatic distress and to effectively reduce the subsequent development of PTSD. Brief CBT also appears to have been more effective than supportive counseling, self-help, repeated assessment, or a naturalistic control group.[196–199]

Treating Acutely Traumatized Children

To date, there are no empirical studies of psychosocial interventions for children and adolescents implemented within the first month after a traumatic event. Nor is there information about the effectiveness of pharmacology or what dosage may be required to be most effective.

Information on the effectiveness of treatment for children is largely based on CBT trials for chronic PTSD. As with adults, there are salient reasons to be concerned about premature interventions with children and adolescents:

1. No empirical evidence exists to support early intervention.
2. There may be developmental reasons to believe that early intervention may be harmful to children at certain ages since it might disrupt the maturation of normal coping and adaptation mechanisms.[200]
3. Since young children base their perceptions of events on their parents' perceptions and behavior (i.e., social referencing), children may perceive that they are still in danger and become more symptomatic if their parents continue to exhibit high levels of post-traumatic distress.

Opiates inhibit neuronal activity in the amygdala and antagonize the actions of CRF and adrenergic neurotransmitters.

One RCT on early intervention with pharmacotherapy involved recently traumatized children on a burn unit with ASD in which the tricyclic antidepressant imipramine produced greater reduction in ASD symptoms than the sedative/hypnotic, chloralhydrate.[201] In a naturalistic study with pediatric burn victims, acute morphine administration during hospitalization prevented the later development of PTSD symptoms.[202]

Pharmacological Treatments and Acute Distress

Given abundant evidence that excessive noradrenergic activity is associated with PTSD, and because it may increase the likelihood of developing intrusive, emotionally arousing memories, one might expect that acute suppression of catecholamines would ameliorate acute post-traumatic distress and prevent PTSD.[141, 195] In the only RCT testing this hypothesis, Pitman et. al. reported promising but somewhat inconclusive results with the adrenergic beta-blocking agent, propranolol, administered to accident victims within six hours of the event.[203] Two other reports also suggest that propranolol may be an effective treatment for acutely traumatized individuals.[204, 205]

Clinical trials are needed for a variety of antiadrenergic, selective serotonergic, and anticonvulsant agents that normalize stress-induced psychological alterations during the acute post-traumatic aftermath.[144, 195]

Key Concepts for Chapter Six:

1. Research indicates that as many as two-thirds of disaster victims never develop PTSD or other psychiatric disorders as a result. Many, however, will experience transient reactions that typically dissipate within a month of the traumatic event and are categorized as acute stress reactions.

2. Acute stress disorder (ASD) is a condition characterized by more dissociative symptoms than avoidant or arousal ones. These symptoms include being focused internally and less aware of external surroundings, having significantly altered perceptions of the external environment (derealization), and having a distorted perception of one's body or identity.

3. Key recommendations for those experiencing acute stress reactions include avoiding re-exposure to traumatic reminders, spending extensive time with supportive friends and family, and patiently allowing normal recovery to occur.

4. Interventions immediately after a traumatic event should include providing for basic needs, orienting one to the disaster and the recovery efforts, reducing psychophysiological arousal, mobilizing support for those most distressed, getting and keeping families together, educating victims about support strategies and resources, and effectively communicating risk without engendering more anxiety.

5. There is no evidence that psychological debriefing is effective. Psychological first aid appears to be a more effective approach during the immediate aftermath of a large-scale traumatic event.

6. Not unlike PTSD treatment efficacy, CBT has proven most effective for those with ASD. Research on pharmacological interventions is at a very preliminary stage.

7. No empirical evidence exists that early intervention is effective with acutely traumatized children; however, there may be a major benefit to ensuring that parents do not experience high levels of post-traumatic distress that could lead children to believe that there is a risk of additional trauma.

Appendix A:
PTSD Assessment Tools for Adults

T HERE is a proliferation of instruments specifically designed for diagnosing PTSD, generally falling into three overlapping categories: assessments of trauma (criterion A_1), diagnostic instruments, or tools that assess PTSD symptom severity (criteria B, C, and D).

Assessment of Exposure to Trauma

Traumatic exposure assessments (see figure A.1 below) fit into two groups: those that inquire about exposure to all possible kinds of traumatic experiences and those that focus on a specific kind of trauma (e.g., child abuse, domestic violence, rape, war-zone exposure, and torture). A more extensive review of adult self-report assessment tools can be found elsewhere.[206]

Typically, instruments used for routine, comprehensive psychological assessment, such as the Million Clinical Multiaxial Inventory (MCMI), Rorschach, or Wechsler Adult Intelligence Scale (WAIS), have not proven useful for diagnosing PTSD. One exception is the Minnesota Multiphasic Personality Inventory (MMPI), which has two, specific subscales for PTSD (see page 85).

Figure A.1   Overview of Trauma Exposure Assessment Tools

	Tool	Self Report	Structured Interview
General	Traumatic Stress Schedule (TSS)	X	
	Potential Stressor Experiences Inventory (PSEI)	X	
	Traumatic Events Questionnaire (TEQ)	X	
	Evaluation of Lifetime Stressors (ELS)	X	X
	The Trauma History Questionnaire (THQ)	X	
	Traumatic Life Events Questionnaire (TLEQ)	X	
	Stressful Life Events Screening Questionnaire (SLESQ)	X	
	Life Stressor Checklist - Revised (LSC-R)	X	
Childhood Trauma	Child Abuse and Trauma Scale	X	
	Childhood Trauma Questionnaire	X	
	Familial Experiences Inventory		X
	Retrospective Assessment of Traumatic Experiences (RATE)	X	
	Early Trauma Inventory (ETI)		X
Domestic Violence	Conflict Tactics Scale (CTS)	X	
	Abusive Behavior Inventory (ABI)	X	
	Sexual Experiences Survey (SES)	X	
	Wyatt Sex History Questionnaire (WSHQ)		X
War Zone Trauma	Combat Exposure Scale (CES)	X	
	Women's Wartime Stressor Scale (WWSS)	X	
Torture	Harvard Trauma Questionnaire (HTQ)	X	

General Traumatic Experiences

Traumatic Stress Schedule (TSS) is a brief, self-report screening questionnaire with good *reliability*. It is quick and easy; however, the TSS has only one question for each of the following traumatic event classes:[207]

1. Robbery
2. Physical assault
3. Sexual assault
4. Loss of a loved one through accident/homicide/suicide
5. Personal injury
6. Serving in combat
7. Property loss due to a disaster or fire
8. Forced evacuation due to imminent danger or environmental hazard
9. Motor vehicle accident causing serious injury
10. Other "terrifying or shocking" experiences

Potential Stressor Experiences Inventory (PSEI) is a self-report scale that measures lifetime exposure to a wide variety of traumatic experiences. It assesses traumatic and non-traumatic events categorized as "high-magnitude" and "low-magnitude" stressors.[208] Since the PSEI obtains information about objective and subjective aspects of traumatic experiences, it is useful for assessing both criterion A_1 and A_2 for each identified event. Finally, the PSEI inquires about the first, most recent, and worst high-magnitude event.

Traumatic Events Questionnaire (TEQ) is a self-report instrument that assesses 11 specific traumatic events.[209] Specific probes inquire about life threat or injury associated with the trauma. It has excellent *test-retest reliability*.

Evaluation of Lifetime Stressors (ELS) was designed as a clinically sensitive instrument that is comprehensive in scope and that optimizes the reporting of traumatic experiences.[210] It is a two-stage instrument, beginning with a self-report questionnaire and ending with a structured interview by a clinician. The ELS was constructed to ask both broad and detailed questions in a clinically sensitive way that does not provoke avoidant behavior or answers that might minimize subject responses on the emotional impact of traumatic experiences.

The Trauma History Questionnaire (THQ) is the most comprehensive instrument.[211] It assesses 24 different types of trauma exposure, some of which would not meet the A_1 criterion, such as expected deaths of loved ones due to natural causes. It functions best as an extensive screening instrument to identify people for more detailed assessment. It has good reliability and

reliability — the extent to which the test produces similar results when administered at different times

test-retest reliability — the extent to which those tested obtain similar scores relative to each other on each administration of the test

validity and has been tested with medical patients, battered women, people with persistent mental illness, and children of holocaust survivors.

Traumatic Life Events Questionnaire (TLEQ) assesses 23 traumatic experiences (including sexual harassment and abortion, that do not meet the A_1 criterion).[212] Its strengths are the probes on the A_2 criterion as well as on physical injury caused by each traumatic event queried.

Stressful Life Events Screening Questionnaire (SLESQ) is a brief screening instrument that assesses 13 items.[213] Its emphasis is more on interpersonal trauma than on disasters. Its focus is exclusively on Criterion A_1 events and not on Criterion A_2 responses. It has been tested on college students and has good psychosomatic properties.

The Life Stressor Checklist-Revised (LSC-R) is a long instrument that inquires about 30 traumatic and non-traumatic stressful events.[214] For each item answered affirmatively, there are two to five, follow-up questions about age, duration, threat appraisal, lifetime impact, and criterion A_2 responses. It has good psychometric properties and has been well accepted by subjects tested.

Specific Traumatic Experiences — Childhood Trauma

Child Abuse and Trauma Scale is a self-report measure for adults that assesses the frequency and intensity of a variety of adverse experiences during childhood and adolescence.[215] It provides a quantitative index of the severity of such experiences. It has been tested on two, large samples of college students and has been shown to have strong *internal consistency.*

Childhood Trauma Questionnaire is a comprehensive self-report scale for adults that assesses four independent factors: physical and emotional abuse, emotional neglect, sexual abuse, and physical neglect.[216] It has high internal consistency and good test-retest reliability.

Familial Experiences Inventory is a comprehensive, clinician-administered diagnostic interview for adults that assesses childhood physical abuse, sexual abuse, and neglect.[217] Information is obtained on each traumatic experience with respect to frequency, severity, duration, and impact.

Retrospective Assessment of Traumatic Experiences (RATE) is a comprehensive instrument.[218] In addition to items on childhood abuse and neglect, it also inquires about parental separation and loss. RATE addresses extra-familial as well as familial abuse. All items are assessed with respect to frequency, intensity, and duration of trauma.

validity — the extent to which the instrument actually measures what it purports to measure

The TLEQ has been standardized on veterans and undergraduate students and has excellent psychometric properties.

The LSC-R is particularly sensitive to stressors affecting women (e.g., one item is about abortion) but can also be used with men.

internal consistency — the degree to which various parts of a test measure the same variables

Early Trauma Inventory (ETI) is a clinical interview to assess childhood emotional, physical, and sexual abuse as well as non-abusive traumas.[219] Formatted like a clinical interview, each subsection begins with an open-ended inquiry about traumatic events, progressing to a series of detailed questions. The ETI is very comprehensive and very detailed.

Specific Trauma Experiences — Domestic Violence

Conflict Tactics Scale (CTS) is one of the first scales of this nature designed to assess partner abuse.[220] It is a self-report subscale on verbal aggression and violence within the family. It has been widely used.

> *The ETI inquires about perpetration, victim age, frequency (at different developmental periods) as well as subjective response at the time of the trauma and at the time of the interview.*

Abusive Behavior Inventory (ABI) accesses (like the CBI) verbal aggression and partner violence as well as physical injury, psychological abuse, and terrorism (without physical assault) within a domestic context.[221] It is a self-report instrument with acceptable reliability and validity.

Sexual Experiences Survey (SES) is a self-report instrument designed to identify rape victims and perpetrators within a normal (in contrast to a treatment-seeking) population.[222] It has good reliability and validity.

Wyatt Sex History Questionnaire (WSHQ) is a structured interview, administered by a clinician, for assessing coercive vs. consensual sexual experiences.[223] One attribute of this instrument is that it has been *standardized* on a multi-ethnic sample of women.

> **standardized** — data collected on a large group and results put in the form of averages by age and group

Specific Trauma Experiences — War-Zone Trauma

Combat Exposure Scale (CES) is a widely used, self-report scale standardized with Vietnam veterans; however, it has been adapted for use with veterans of other conflicts (e.g., Persian Gulf War, Somalia, Bosnia).[224] It has good internal consistency and test-retest reliability.

Women's Wartime Stressor Scale (WWSS) is a self-report instrument to assess unique aspects of war zone exposure relevant to the experience of female Vietnam veterans.[225] In addition to traditional war zone items, this scale also assesses sexual trauma and nursing-related events. It has good *psychometric properties*.

> **psychometric properties** — the elements of constructing a useful instrument such as establishing reliability and validity

Specific Trauma Experiences — Torture

Harvard Trauma Questionnaire (HTQ) assesses torture, trauma, and PTSD among Indo-Chinese refugees.[226] It is a culturally sensitive, self-report instrument that has both open-ended and detailed questions in which respondents report on their own worst experiences as well as about torture experiences that they witnessed or heard about.

Diagnostic Instruments

Diagnostic scales are either in the form of structured clinical interviews administered by a clinician or lay interviews designed for epidemiological research. A number of self-report, PTSD symptom severity scores (see pages 85 through 86) are sometimes used for diagnostic purposes, as well. Those with higher scores may be considered to have PTSD; however, in general, it is better to conduct a systematic diagnostic assessment. The Clinician-Administered PTSD Scale (CAPS), designed by the National Center for PTSD, functions as both a diagnostic and symptom-severity instrument.

Structured Clinical Interview for DSM-IV (SCID): PTSD Module[227]

The SCID provides a comprehensive DSM-IV diagnostic assessment with a separate module for each Axis I disorder. Therefore, it is not only useful for diagnosing PTSD, but also for diagnosing any possible comorbid disorders. Trained clinicians must administer the SCID since it is a structured interview with a number of probes designed to elicit relevant clinical information. Used widely and demonstrating good performance, the major limitation of SCID is that it only provides dichotomous (Yes/No) information about the presence or absence of each symptom. Though it determines the nature of a traumatic experience, it does not measure the severity of such exposure. Therefore, although the SCID is the gold standard for diagnostic assessment, it can neither provide information about symptom severity, nor can it detect any changes in symptom severity following treatment.

Clinician Administered PTSD Scale (CAPS)[228]

Designed as a quantitative expansion of the PTSD module of the SCID, CAPS is a structured interview administered by a trained clinician. Criteria A_1 and A_2 are assessed before inquiring about B, C, and D symptoms. Like the SCID, CAPS provides information on both current and lifetime PTSD. Unlike the SCID, it provides a continuous measure of each PTSD (and associated) symptom along two dimensions: intensity and frequency. Therefore, the total PTSD severity score is the sum of the separate intensity and frequency scores. CAPS monitors the response to treatment and is the instrument of choice in drug or psychotherapy treatment research. It has excellent psychometric properties.

PTSD-Interview[229]

This is a diagnostic instrument that also measures the severity of PTSD symptoms. It differs from the previously mentioned assessment tools because of lay administration. Subjects, rather than the clinician, rate their own symptom severity. Thus, it is more a self-report instrument than a structured interview, more closely resembling the CIDI (see below).

Diagnostic instruments include:
- ▶ *Structured Clinical Interview for DSM-IV (SCID): PTSD module*
- ▶ *Clinician Administered PTSD Scale (CAPS)*
- ▶ *PTSD-Interview*
- ▶ *The Davidson Self-Rating PTSD Scale*
- ▶ *Composite International Diagnostic Interview (CIDI)*
- ▶ *The Post-traumatic Stress Diagnostic Scale (PDS)*

The SCID provides information about the presence of both current or lifetime diagnoses so that it can be determined whether someone who currently does not meet DSM-IV criteria for PTSD may have done so at some time in the past.

A growing trend has been to substitute the CAPS for the SCID: PTSD Module, which facilitates simultaneous PTSD diagnostic assessment and symptom severity measurement.

The Davidson Self-Rating PTSD Scale[230]

This 17-item, self-report measure derives from DSM-IV-defined PTSD symptom clusters. The scale rates each item from 0 to 4 for both frequency and severity during the past week. The total scale has demonstrated good test-retest reliability and internal consistency. The subscales also have high reliability in diagnosing PTSD compared to the SCID.

Composite International Diagnostic Interview (CIDI)[231]

This is a structured diagnostic interview designed for survey research employing lay rather than clinician interviewers for assessing all DSM-IV diagnoses. The PTSD module has good *sensitivity* and *specificity*. Used in the National Comorbidity Study, the CIDI currently is the instrument of choice for epidemiologic research concerning PTSD.

sensitivity — percent of cases correctly identified by the instrument

specificity — percent of non-cases correctly identified by the instrument

The Post-traumatic Stress Diagnostic Scale (PDS)[232]

Evolved from the PSS (see below) for better diagnostic specificity, the PDS begins with a brief assessment of traumatic exposure followed by the 17 DSM-IV (TR) PTSD symptoms that are scored on a four-point scale that focuses on symptom frequency during the past month. Functional impairments are assessed by nine additional items. Its test-retest reliability, internal consistency, sensitivity, and specificity are excellent. It has shown excellent agreement with the SCID, yielding the same diagnosis 82 percent of the time.

Diagnostic Interview Schedule IV (DIS-IV)

The DIS-IV is a structured diagnostic interview (like the CIDI) designed to be administered by experienced lay interviewers without clinical training.[233] It has been used in psychiatric survey research for decades to assess the prevalence of psychiatric disorders in the general population. Although it has been displaced in some quarters by the CIDI, it is still an excellent instrument. The PTSD module of the DIS-IV has good sensitivity and specificity. [234]

PTSD Symptom Severity Scales

For some of the following scales, cut-points have been established, above which a PTSD diagnosis is likely.

PTSD Checklist (PCL)[235]

This self-report questionnaire assesses 17 DSM-IV (TR) PTSD symptoms on a five-point scale. It has good sensitivity and specificity, and it correlates well with other standard measures. Although it was initially used mostly in research with combat veterans, it has performed well, more recently, in numerous civilian settings.

PTSD Symptom Scale (PSS)[236]

This self-report questionnaire assesses the 17 DSM-IV (TR) PTSD symptoms on a four-point scale. It has excellent psychometric properties and has been used mostly with rape victims.

PK-Scale of the MMPI-2[237]

This consists of a 49-item subscale of the MMPI-2. Although mostly used with veterans, it has also performed well with rape victims and other traumatized groups. It *correlates* well with the CAPS. Its advantage is that, since it is a subscale of the MMPI, it can be extracted from the entire scale when the MMPI-2 is administered routinely. Its possible disadvantage is that it is a long scale and has not always performed as well as other instruments for assessing PTSD symptom severity.

PS-Scale of the MMPI-2[238]

Like the PK Scale, this was originally developed for epidemiological research with Vietnam veterans. It may have broader applicability to other traumatized groups (e.g., child abuse, criminal victimization) but has only moderate *predictive validity* and has not been studied extensively.

SCL-PTSD[239, 240]

This 28-item scale was extracted from the *Symptom Checklist-90 (SCL-90)*. The SCL-PTSD was standardized on women with a history of criminal victimization. It is not as well validated as some of the other scales, but its advantage (like the PK and PS Scales of the MMPI-2) is that it was extracted from an assessment instrument that is widely used.

Impact of Event Scale-Revised (IES-R)[241]

This revision of a self-report scale (widely used in PTSD assessment) consists of 22 items that tap criteria B, C, and D symptoms, each of which are rated on a five-point scale. It was originally tested on natural disaster survivors and has performed quite well.

Symptom severity scales include:

▶ *PTSD Checklist (PCL)*

▶ *PTSD Symptom Scale (PSS)*

▶ *PK and PS Scales of the MMPI-2*

▶ *SCL-PTSD*

▶ *Impact of Event Scale-Revised (IES-R))*

▶ *Mississippi Scale for Combat-Related PTSD (M-PTSD)*

▶ *Revised Civilian Mississippi Scale*

▶ *Penn Inventory*

▶ *Trauma Symptom Checklist-40 (TSC-40)*

▶ *Trauma Symptom Inventory (TSI)*

correlates — the degree to which two scores systematically relate to one another

predictive validity — the extent to which scores on an instrument are predictive of actual performance

Symptom Checklist-90 (SCL-90) — a broad-spectrum instrument that assesses many different psychological domains, including depressive, psychotic, and anxiety symptoms

Mississippi Scale for Combat-Related PTSD (M-PTSD)[242]

This is a 35-item instrument that, in addition to criterion B, C, and D symptoms, taps associated symptoms such as guilt and suicidality. It has performed extremely well in research and clinical settings. The M-PTSD was developed and standardized with combat veterans.

Revised Civilian Mississippi Scale[243]

Modified from the M-PTSD and designed for non-veterans, this scale has been used mostly with civilian survivors of natural disasters. The quality of reliability and validity results have been mixed with this assessment instrument.

Penn Inventory[244]

Developed and validated on both veterans and civilian disaster survivors, this 26-item scale has exhibited high sensitivity and specificity despite the lack of extensive testing.

Trauma Symptom Checklist-40 (TSC-40)[245]

Developed for use with adult survivors of childhood sexual abuse, the TSC-20 subscales tap anxiety, depression, dissociation, post sexual abuse trauma, and sleep disturbance. TSC-20 has been used mostly with young adults and has performed well.

Trauma Symptom Inventory (TSI)[246]

The TSI expands the TSC-40 to a 100-item instrument with 10 subscales that tap anxiety, depression, anger, PTSD symptoms, sexual concerns/behavior, and dissociation. It correlates well with other PTSD scales and has been useful as both a clinical and research tool.

Appendix B:
PTSD Assessment Tools for Children

As with adults, scales for the assessment and diagnosis of PTSD in children can be divided into the three overlapping categories presented in appendix A:

1. Assessment of trauma (Criterion A_1)
2. Diagnostic instruments
3. Assessment of PTSD symptom severity

Scales for children must be developmentally sensitive and must be worded so that they can be comprehended accurately. Scales for children often have companion scales for parents or teachers. Finally, it is inadvisable to administer questionnaires to children younger than six, since they lack the verbal and cognitive abstracting ability to understand questions and to respond appropriately.

More detailed information on all of these scales can be found in Kathleen Nader's excellent recent chapter on assessing traumatic experiences in children.[247]

Assessment of Trauma (Criterion A_1)

My Worst Experience Survey (MWES) and My Worst School Experience Survey (MWSES)[248]

These are both lengthy interviews that must be administered by a skilled clinician. They assess the child's most stressful experience either in the general environment or specifically in the school setting. Such stressors include abuse, assault, disaster, death of loved ones, parental separation, or family problems. The interview also inquires systematically about emotional response to such stressors so that criterion A_2 can also be assessed.

Traumatic Event Screening Instrument for Children (TESI-C)[249]

The TESI has child and parent (TESI-C and TESI-P) versions. It is a 15-item, broad-spectrum interview that must be administered by a trained clinician. The TESI inquires about accidents, disasters, hospitalizations, physical abuse, sexual abuse, and exposure to domestic or other violent events. Still being developed, it has not been subjected to validity or reliability testing.

When Bad Things Happen Scale (WBTHS)[259]

This is a self-report diagnostic instrument that has four associated scales, one of which, the "Dimensions of Stressful Events (DOSE)" measures Criterion A events. (The other accompanying scales involve an interview with the child, a parent interview, and a parent questionnaire regarding the child.) WBTHS has been used with Armenian, Israeli, and American children. Preliminary data suggest that it has good validity and reliability.

Computer programs for scoring and analyzing the WBTH are available through the World Health Organization (WHO) and Centers for Disease Control (CDC).[247] (pp. 317–318)

Children's Sexual Behavior Inventory 3 (CSBI-3)[251]

CSBI-3 has been translated into French, Spanish, German, and Swedish.

This simply worded, 36-item questionnaire can be administered by parents or primary caregivers. CSBI-3 assesses the frequency of a wide variety of sexual behaviors on a four-point scale, including traumatic and non-traumatic (e.g., self-stimulation and voluntary activities with others). Research with the CSBI-3 indicates that it can distinguish sexually abused from non-abused children. Its recommended best use is "as part of a comprehensive evaluation . . . with careful clinical interviewing and assessment of other behavior problems."[247] (page 335)

Child Rating Scales of Exposure to Interpersonal Abuse (CRS-EIA) and the Angie/Andy CRS (A/A CRS)[247 (pp. 321–325), 252, 253]

These are clinician-administered scales to assess the frequency and severity of exposure to interpersonal abuse by 6-11 year olds. The questionnaires consist of cartoons depicting sexual abuse, physical abuse, or witnessing family/community violence. The A/A CRS is designed for girls (Angie) and boys (Andy) so that the cartoons are gender appropriate for the child being assessed. There is also a companion A/A PRS for parents, which is keyed to the A/A CRS that has verbal items rather than cartoons. The instrument for parents is still being revised but has performed well in preliminary trials and is proposed for assessing complex PTSD as well as DSM-IV (TR) PTSD.

Diagnostic Instruments

As with adults, these include structured clinical interviews to be administered by a clinician or lay interviews designed for epidemiological research. Self-report symptom severity scales (see pages 85–86) are also sometimes used for diagnostic purposes. Again, as with adults, the Clinician Administered PTSD Scale [for children (CAPS-C)] was designed as both a diagnostic and symptom-severity scale.

Diagnostic Interview for Children and Adolescents-Revised (DICA-R)[242 (pp. 319-320), 254]

inter-rater reliability — the degree to which different raters agree on a diagnosis based on the use of the instrument

The DICA-R is the child equivalent of the SCID (see appendix A). It is a broad-spectrum diagnostic interview designed to assess all DSM-IV diagnoses with a specific module dedicated to PTSD. There is a four-point rating for symptom severity that focuses on frequency rather than intensity. The PTSD module has good *inter-rater reliability,* but its performance has been mixed with regard to specificity and sensitivity. Training is required to administer this instrument properly.

Clinician Administered
PTSD Scale for Children (CAPS-C)[247 (pp. 307–309), 255]

This is the child equivalent of the CAPS (see appendix A). It is a structured interview that assesses the severity (e.g., intensity plus frequency) of each PTSD symptom. Psychometric testing has yet to be conducted. There is a manual that accompanies the CAPS-C, and clinicians must receive training to use it.

Diagnostic Interview Schedule
for Children, version 2.3 (DISC)[247 (pp. 321–322), 256]

This DISC has been designed for epidemiological research (like the DIS-IV for adults — see appendix A). It has both child and parent versions. Preliminary results suggest that the PTSD module of the DISC may not have sufficient specificity and sensitivity to detect PTSD in community surveys.

Children's PTSD Inventory (CPTSDI)[257–259]

This is a clinician-administered structural interview for children and adolescents aged 7 to 18. It measures trauma exposure, PTSD symptoms, and functional impairment and has been used extensively due to its excellent reliability and validity.

PTSD Symptom Severity Scales

UCLA PTSD Reaction Index
for DSM-IV (UCLA-PTSD-RI)[247 (pp. 309–312), 257, 260]

This is one of the best-validated instruments in PTSD research with children and adolescents aged 6 to 17. It takes 20 to 30 minutes to administer and consists of three parts: Part I is a brief lifetime trauma screen; Part II evaluates objective and subjective aspects of exposure to a traumatic event; and Part III consists of 22 questions rated on a five-point scale regarding the frequency of post-traumatic symptoms. The UCLA-PTSD-RI has good reliability and validity.

Child's Reaction to
Traumatic Events Scale (CRTES)[247 (pp. 312–313), 261]

CRTES is a revision of the Impact of Events Scale modified for children (see appendix A). It focuses on PTSD symptoms of intrusions and avoidance but not hyperarousal symptoms. It is a brief, 15-item scale that is easy to administer. The CRTES is currently undergoing psychometric evaluation.

As with adults, a typical practice in clinical assessment or research with children might be to use the DICA-R to determine comorbid diagnoses (because the PTSD module of the DICA-R lacks diagnostic sensitivity and specificity) and to substitute the CAPS-C for the DICA-R PTSD module for simultaneous PTSD diagnostic assessment and symptom severity measurement.

Considered an excellent instrument for assessing PTSD severity, the UCLA-PTSD-RI has been successfully administered to a variety of traumatized populations and translated into several languages. It has performed well in research with children exposed to natural disasters, war, and schoolyard sniper attacks.

Children's Impact of Traumatic Events Scale (CITES)[247 (pp. 328–331), 262, 263]

This 78-item measure with four subscales — PTSD, Social Relations, Abuse Attributions, and Eroticism — is a clinician-administered, semi-structured interview that assesses symptoms on a three-point scale. Correlations with other child abuse scales have been mixed. This may be because the CITES expands the inquiry beyond conventional, post-abuse outcomes to assess social reactions and other subjective responses often exhibited by sexually abused children.

Trauma Symptom Checklist for Children (TSCC)[264, 265]

This is a 54-item, self-report questionnaire for 8 to 16 year olds that assesses the effects of trauma with respect to PTSD, anxiety, depression, anger, and dissociation. It has good internal consistency and validity, is easy-to-use, and cost effective. Non-traumatized children can complete the TSCC within 20 minutes (traumatized children often require more time).

The Child PTSD Symptom Scale (CPSS)[257, 266]

The CPSS is a new scale with only preliminary psychometric evaluation, but initial results are quite promising.

The CPSS is modified from the PTSD Symptom Scale (see appendix A). In addition to assessing the frequency of PTSD symptoms, it also has seven questions on social, school, and other functional domains.

Child Report of Post-Traumatic Symptoms/Parent Report of Post-Traumatic Symptoms (CROPS/PROPS)[267, 268]

CROPS/PROPS assesses a broad range of post-traumatic symptoms from both the child's and parents' perspectives. Early testing has focused on urban and rural children in grades three through eight. Only preliminary psychometric data are currently available.

Child Dissociative Checklist (CDC)[247 (pp. 325–328), 269]

This is a 20-item, easily administered instrument designed to assess dissociative symptoms in sexually abused children, such as:

- ▶ Dissociative amnesia
- ▶ Rapid shifts in observable cognitive/behavioral indices
- ▶ Spontaneous trance states
- ▶ Hallucinations
- ▶ Alterations in identity
- ▶ Aggressive/sexual behavior

It has excellent internal consistency and test-retest reliability, and training is not required to administer the CDC. It has proven to be a cost-effective and useful instrument for detecting dissociative symptoms in children and adolescents.

Appendix C:
ASD Assessment Tools

MANY of the scales described in appendices A and B are useful for assessing ASD as well. The following reviews these overlaps among tools for assessment of trauma, diagnostic instruments, and symptom severity scales.

Assessment of Trauma

Since criteria A_1 and A_2 are the same for both diagnoses, many of the scales described previously for PTSD are applicable to assessment of ASD. The major exception would be an instrument that assesses trauma of long duration, such as sexual/physical abuse in children. Instruments for combat/war zone stress or torture would also not be useful in ASD assessment unless they were administered shortly after exposure to the specific traumatic event that precipitated ASD symptoms. This is because ASD can only be diagnosed within one month of initial exposure to the traumatic experience in question.

The following trauma scales are useful for ASD assessment in adults:

- TSS: Traumatic Stress Schedule
- PSEI: Potential Stressor Experiences Inventory
- TEQ: Traumatic Events Questionnaire
- THQ: Trauma History Questionnaire
- SLESQ: Stressful Life Events Screening Questionnaire
- CTS: Conflict Tactics Scale
- ABI: Abusive Behavior Inventory
- SES: Sexual Experiences Survey
- WSHQ: Wyatt Sex History Questionnaire
- HTQ: Harvard Trauma Questionnaire

Under certain conditions, the Combat Exposure Scale (CES) and the Women's Wartime Stressor Scale (WWSS) can be helpful. Additionally, the Harvard Trauma Questionnaire (HTQ) has been used in many cross-cultural settings, whereas the CES and WWSS have been used primarily with European and American subjects.

Questionnaires designed for adults concerning childhood trauma would not be useful in ASD; however, all trauma scales described in appendix B would be useful for ASD assessment, if such trauma occurred within one month of the interview.

Diagnostic Instruments

The ASD modules of the SCID and CIDI could be used for diagnostic assessment in adults (see appendix A).[227, 231] The ASD modules of the DICA-R and DISC could be used for diagnosing ASD in children (see appendix B).[254, 256]

Symptom Severity Scales

None of the symptom severity scales described for adults (appendix A) or children (appendix B) could be used for ASD since these scales lack the dissociative items and overemphasize the intrusion/avoidant/hyperarousal symptom presentation needed for ASD assessment.

Three scales have been developed for ASD assessment; however, they have only been used with adults.

1. **Acute Stress Disorder Interview (ASDI)**[271] — ASDI consists of 19 "yes/no" questions organized within ASD diagnostic symptom clusters: five on dissociation, four on reexperiencing, four on avoidance, and six on arousal. ASD severity is determined simply by summing up the affirmative answers (one point for each). ASDI has good internal consistency, test-retest reliability, sensitivity, and specificity.

2. **Acute Stress Disorder Scale (ASDS)**[272] — ASDS substitutes a five-point, Likert scale for each of the 19 items included in the ASDI. Therefore, it provides better fine-grained assessment of ASD symptom severity, analogous to the PCL and PSS for PTSD. It has good sensitivity, specificity, and test-retest reliability. As with the ASDI, the ASDS does not adequately predict later development of PTSD.[272]

3. **Stanford Acute Stress Reaction Questionnaire (SASRQ)**[273] — SASRQ is the first measure developed for assessing ASD and has undergone several revisions. A 30-item, six-point, self-report Likert scale inventory inquires about dissociative, reexperiencing, somatic, hyperarousal, insomnia, and cognitive symptoms. Earlier versions had good internal consistency for dissociative and anxiety symptoms; however, diagnostic validity and ability to predict subsequent PTSD has not been proven.

A more extensive review of these scales can be found in *Assessing Psychological Trauma and PTSD, Second Edition.*[270]

Glossary

A

adrenergic response — neuronal activation mediated by either norepinephrine (noradrenaline) or epinephrine (adrenaline)

affect lability — rapid and unpredictable shifts in mood state

amnesia — mental syndrome characterized by partial or complete memory loss

amygdala — principal nucleus in the brain for appraising emotional input and threatening stimuli and then mobilizing protective, defensive, or escape behavior

anxiolytics — medications that relieve anxiety

ataques de nervios — a common symptom of distress among Hispanic American groups involving anxiety, uncontrollable shouting and crying, trembling, heart palpitations, difficulty breathing, dizziness, fainting spells, and dissociative symptoms (e.g., amnesia and alteration of consciousness)

B

benzodiazepine family of drugs — a very effective and widely prescribed class of medications for anxiety that includes: diazepam, lorazepam, alprazolam, and clonazepam

borderline personality disorder — a personality disorder characterized by extreme instabilities fluctuating between normal functioning and psychic disability

C

calor — a stress-related syndrome observed among Salvadoran women described as a surge of intense heat that may rapidly spread throughout the entire body for a few moments or for several days

cognitive-behavioral approaches — therapeutic approaches that focus on patterns of reinforcement, learning and conditioning models, and correcting erroneous cognitions

comorbid disorders — major psychiatric disorders that are present at the same time an individual has full-fledged PTSD

correlates — the degree to which two scores systematically relate to one another

cortisol — a hormone that increases energy by raising blood glucose levels, decreases immune processes, and causes other metabolic and neurobiological actions

countertransference — the clinician's psychological reaction to something the patient said or did

D

depersonalization — an alteration in the perception or experience of the self so that one feels detached from, and as if one is an outside observer of, one's mental processes or body (e.g., feeling like one is in a dream)

derealization — an alteration in the perception or experience of the external world so that it seems strange or unreal (e.g., people may seem unfamiliar or mechanical)

dissociation — an abnormal cognitive/emotional state in which one's perception of oneself, one's environment, or the relationship between oneself and one's environment is altered significantly

dissociative identity disorder — previously called multiple personality disorder, which is characterized by one's personality becoming so fragmented that pronounced changes in behavior and reactivity are noticed between different social situations or social roles

E

extapyramidal — uncontrollable involuntary motor movements or excessive rigidity

F

fragmented thoughts — the inability to sustain continuity and coherence in one's cognitive processes

G

generalized anxiety disorder — a psychiatric disorder marked by unrealistic worry, apprehension, and uncertainty as well as physical symptoms, such as: muscle tension, restlessness, dry mouth, and frequent urination

H

hallucination — a compelling perceptual experience of seeing, hearing, or smelling something that is not actually present

hematopoietic — suppression of the bone marrow's capacity to produce red and white blood cells

hyper-reactive psychophysiological state — a state in which emotions are heightened and aroused and even minor events may produce a state in which the heart pounds rapidly, muscles are tense, and there is great, overall agitation

hypervigilance — preoccupied by watchful or protective behavior motivated by excessive fears for personal safety

hypothalamic-pituitary-adrenocortical (HPA) axis — three anatomic structures that participate collectively in the hormonal response to stress: the hypothalamus (in the brain), the pituitary gland, and the outer layer (cortex) of the adrenal gland

I

imaginal exposure — systematically assisting trauma survivors to confront distressing trauma memories though the use of mental imagery

internal consistency — the degree to which various parts of a test measure the same variables

inter-rater reliability — the degree to which different raters agree on a diagnosis based on the use of the instrument

in-vivo exposure — patients practice techniques learned in therapy in the environment that represents their most-feared situation

L

lifetime PTSD — those who developed PTSD at any time in their lives

N

neurotransmitters — chemical messengers that transmit signals from one nerve cell to another to elicit physiological responses

neutrality — a psychoanalytic technique by which clinicians reveal as little of themselves as possible so that thoughts, memories, and feelings generated during therapy come from the patient's intrapsychic processes rather than from an interpersonal relationship between patient and clinician

P

panic disorder — a psychiatric disorder marked by intense anxiety and panic as well as many physical symptoms, such as: palpitations, shortness of breath, dizziness, sweating, and a sense of impending death

pathological changes — changes resulting in an abnormal condition that prevents proper psychological functioning

peritraumatic dissociation — dissociation during and shortly after the trauma

personality pathology — maladaptive pattern of relating to other people that severely impairs social functioning and adaptive potential

pharmacological probe — a drug that can activate psychobiological mechanisms involved in the stress response

physiological reactivity — quickening of the heart rate, blood pressure, and breathing, resulting from exposure to internal or external cues that symbolize or resemble an aspect of the traumatic event

physioneurosis — a label for the clinically significant physiological as well as psychological changes believed to be part of the "war neurosis" syndrome

play therapy — a technique for treating young children in which they reveal their problems on a fantasy level with dolls, clay, and other toys

post-synaptic neuron — the downstream neuron that is the target of neurotransmission

predictive validity — the extent to which scores on an instrument are predictive of actual performance

pre-synaptic neuron — the neuron that initiates neurotransmission by releasing the neurotransmitter into the synaptic cleft

psychic balance — a dynamic equilibrium state between those thoughts, feelings, memories, and urges the conscious can tolerate and those it cannot

psychic numbing — the inability to feel any emotions, either positive (love and pleasure) or negative (fear or guilt), also described as an "emotional anesthesia"

psychodynamic approaches — therapeutic approaches that focus on unconscious and conscious motivations and drives

psychogenic amnesia — the inability to remember emotionally charged events for psychological rather than neurological reasons

psychological debriefing — an intervention conducted by trained professionals shortly after a catastrophe, allowing victims to talk about their experience and receive information on "normal" types of reactions to such an event

psychological first aid — an approach designed to ameliorate immediate post-traumatic distress based on the expectation that every survivor, no matter how upset, will achieve normal recovery

psychological probe — a visual or auditory stimulus reminiscent of a traumatic experience to which a person with PTSD is exposed

psychometric instruments — tests that measure psychological factors, such as personality, intelligence, beliefs, and fears

psychometric properties — the elements of constructing a useful instrument such as establishing reliability and validity

R

receptors — membrane-bound protein molecules with a highly specific shape that facilitate binding by neurotransmitters or medications

reliability — the extent to which the test produces similar results when administered at different times

repression — a hypothetical, unconscious process by which unacceptable (often trauma-related) thoughts and feelings are kept out of conscious awareness

S

saccadic eye movements — rapid intermittent eye movement, such as that which occurs when the eyes fix on one point after another in the visual field

schizophrenia — a major psychiatric disorder characterized by disorganization and fragmentation of thought, delusions, hallucinations, apathy, disturbance of language and communication, and withdrawal from social interaction

secondary traumatization — feelings, personal distress, and symptoms sometimes evoked in people who live with an individual with PTSD

self-cohesion — knowledge and integration of previously unconscious motivations

sensitivity — percent of cases correctly identified by the instrument

somatization — the expression of emotional distress through physical symptoms such as peptic ulcer, asthma, or chronic pain

specificity — percent of non-cases correctly identified by the instrument

standardized — data collected on a large group and results put in the form of averages by age and group

startle reactions — "jumpy" behavior manifested as a tendency to exhibit an exaggerated startle response to unexpected noises or movements by others

Subjective Units of Distress Scale — a scale ranging from 10–100 with 10 being the least anxiety provoking and 100 being the most anxiety provoking. The SUDS scoring system allows the patient to express exactly how upsetting or distressing certain stimuli are in comparison to other anxiety experiences

sympathetic nervous system — part of the autonomic nervous system that regulates arousal functions such as heart rate and blood flow

Symptom Checklist-90 (SCL-90) — is a broad-spectrum instrument that assesses many different psychological domains, including depressive, psychotic, and anxiety symptoms

synaptic cleft — the space between one neuron and the next that must be traversed by neurotransmitters

T

teratogenic — producing fetal abnormalities during pregnancy

test-retest reliability — the extent to which those tested obtain similar scores relative to each other on each administration of the test

V

validity — the extent to which the instrument actually measures what it purports to measure

vicarious traumatization — feelings, personal distress, and symptoms that are sometimes evoked in clinicians working with PTSD patients

W

well encapsulated — psychological buffers that prevent a person from experiencing current distress from a previous traumatic event

References

1. Kessler, R.C., Sonnega, A., Bromet, E., Hughes, M., Nelson, C.B. (1995). Posttraumatic stress disorder in the National Comorbidity Survey. *Arch Gen Psychiatry, 52*: 1048-1060.

2. De Jong, J.T.V.M., Komproe, I.H., Van Ommeren, M., El Masri, M., Mesfin, A., Khaled, N., van de Put, W.A.M., & Somasundaram, D. (2001). Lifetime events and posttraumatic stress disorder in 4 postconflict settings. *Journal of the American Medical Association, 286*, 555-562.

3. American Psychiatric Committee on Nomenclature and Statistics ed. (1980). *Diagnostic and Statistical Manual of Mental Disorders, Third Edition*. Washington, DC: American Psychiatric Association.

4. American Psychiatric Committee on Nomenclature and Statistics ed. (1994). *Diagnostic and Statistical Manual of Mental Disorders, Fourth Edition*. Washington, DC: American Psychiatric Association.

5. American Psychiatric Association (2000). *Diagnostic and statistical manual of mental disorders, 4th ed. Text revision*. Washington, DC: American Psychiatric Association.

6. Mueser, K. Personal Communication. June 26, 2003.

7. van der Kolk, B.A., Weisaeth, L., van der Hart, O. (1996). History of trauma in psychiatry. In B.A. van der Kolk, A.C., McFarlane & L. Weisaeth (Eds.), *Traumatic stress: The effects of overwhelming experience on mind, body, and society*. New York/London: Guilford Press, 47-74.

8. Cohen, M.E., White, P.D., Johnson, R.E. (1948). Neurocirculatory asthenia, anxiety neurosis, or the effort syndrome. *Arch Intern Med, 81*: 260-281.

9. Trimble, M.R. (1985). Post-traumatic stress disorder: History of a concept. In C.R. Figley (Ed.), *Trauma and its wake: Volume 1: The study and treatment of post-traumatic stress disorder*. New York: Burnner/Mazel; 5-14.

10. Kardiner, A. (1941). *The traumatic neurosis of war*. New York: Hoeber.

11. Schnurr, P.P. (1991). PTSD and combat-related psychiatric symptoms in older veterans. *PTSD Research Quarterly, 2*: 1-6.

12. Schnurr, P.P., & Green, B.L. (Eds.) (2004). *Trauma and health: Physical health consequences of exposure to extreme stress*. Washington, DC: American Psychological Association.

13. Harvey, A.G., Bryant, R.A. (1998). Acute stress disorder after mild traumatic brain injury. *Journal of Nervous and Mental Disorders, 186*, 333-337.

14. Green, B.L., Friedman, M.J., de Jong, J., Solomon, S., Keane, T., Fairbank, J.A., Donelan, B., & Frey-Wouters, E. (2003). *Trauma interventions in war and peace: Prevention, practice, and policy*. Amsterdam: Kluwer Academic/Plenum.

15. Friedman, M.J. (2002). Future pharmacotherapy for post-traumatic stress disorder: Prevention and treatment. *Psychiatric Clinics of North America, 25*, 427-441.

16. Friedman, M.J., & Rosenheck, R.A. (1996). PTSD as a persistent mental illness. In: Soreff, S., ed. *The seriously and persistently mentally ill: The state-of-the-art treatment handbook* (pp. 369-389). Seattle, WA: Hogrefe & Huber.

17. Brewin, C.R., Andrews, B., & Valentine, J.D. (2000). Meta-analysis of risk factors for posttraumatic stress disorder in trauma-exposed adults. *Journal of Consulting and Clinical Psychology, 68*, 748-766.

18. Fairbank, J.A., Schlenger, W.E., Saigh, P.A., Davidson, J.R.T. (1995). An epidemiologic profile of post-traumatic stress disorder: Prevalence, comorbidity, and risk factors. In: Friedman, M.J., Charney, D.S., Deutch, A.Y., eds. *Neurobiological and clinical consequences of stress: From normal adaptation to post-traumatic stress disorder*. Philadelphia, PA: Lippincott-Raven; 415-427.

19. Caspi, A., Sugden, K., Moffitt, T.E., Taylor, A., Craig, I.W., Harrington, H., McClay, J., Mill, J., Martin, J., Braithwaite, A., & Poulton, R. (2003). Influence of life stress on depression: Moderation by a polymorphism in the 5HTT gene. *Science, 301*, 386-389.

20. True, W., & Pitman, R.K. (1999). Genetics and posttraumatic stress disorder. In P.A. Saigh & J.D. Bremner (Eds.), *Posttraumatic stress disorder: A comprehensive text* (pp. 144-159). Boston: Allyn & Bacon.

21. Wilson, J.P., Keane, T.M. (Eds.) (2004). *Assessing psychological trauma and PTSD, Second Edition*. New York: Guilford.

22. Friedman, M.J., & McEwen, B. (2004). PTSD, health, and allostatic load? In P.P. Schnurr & B.L. Green (Eds.), *Trauma and health: Physical health consequences of exposure to extreme stress.* (pp 157-188), Washington, DC: American Psychological Association.

23. Schnurr, P.P., Friedman, M.J., & Rosenberg, S.D. (1993). Premilitary MMPI scores as predictors of combat-related PTSD symptoms. *Am J Psychiatry, 150,* 479-483.

24. Stein, M.B., Walker, J.R., Hazen, A.L., & Forde, D.R. (1997). Full and partial posttraumatic stress disorder: Findings from a community survey. *Am J Psychiatry, 154,* 1114-1119.

25. Weiss, D.S., Marmar, C.R., Schlenger, W.E., Fairbank, J.A., Jordan, B.K., Hough, R.L., et al., (1992). The prevalence of lifetime and partial post-traumatic stress disorder in Vietnam theater veterans. *J Trauma Stress, 5,* 365-376.

26. Herman, J.L. (1992). Complex PTSD: A syndrome in survivors of prolonged and repeated trauma. *J Traumatic Stress, 5*: 377-391.

27. Linehan, M.M., Tutek, D.A., Heard, H.L., Armstrong, H.E. (1994). Interpersonal outcome of cognitive behavioral treatment for chronically suicidal borderline patients. *American Journal of Psychiatry, 151,* 1771-1776.

28. Lindy, J.D. (1993). Focal psychoanalytic psychotherapy. In J.P. Wilson, & B. Raphael (Eds.), *The international handbook of traumatic stress syndromes.* New York, Plenum Press.

29. Horowitz, M.J. (1986). *Stress response syndromes (2nd Edition).* New York, Jason Aronson.

30. Foa, E.B. & Rothbaum, B.O. (1997). *Treating the trauma of rape: A cognitive-behavioral therapy for PTSD.* New York, Guilford.

31. Foa, E.B., Keane, T.M., & Friedman, M.J. (2000). *Practice Guidelines for PTSD.* New York, Guilford.

32. Ursano, R.J., Bell, C.C., Eth, S, Friedman, M.J., Norwood, A.E., Pfefferbaum, B., Pynoos, R.S, Zatzick, D.F., Benedek, D.M., McIntyre, J.S., Charles, S.C., Altshuler, K., Cook, I., Cross, C.D., Mellman, L., Moench, L.A., Norquist, G.S., Twemlow, S.W., Woods, S., Yager, J. (2004). American Psychiatric Association Work Group on ASD and PTSD; American Psychiatric Association Steering Committee on Practice Guidelines. *Practice Guidelines for the treatment of acute stress and post-traumatic stress disorder.* Washington: American Psychiatric Association

33. *The VA/DoD Clinical Practice Guidelines for the Management of Post-Traumatic Stress* (2004). Washington, DC, U.S. Departments of Veterans Affairs and Defense. Retrieved from http://www.oqp.med.va.gov/ cpg/PTS/PTS_base.htm.

34. Rothbaum, B.O., Foa, E.G., Davidson, J.R.T., Cahill, S.P., Comptom, J., Connor, K.M., Aston, M., Berkebile, N., (2004). *Augmentation of sertraline with prolonged exposure in PTSD.* Poster presented at the 159th Annual Meeting, American Psychological Association, New York, NY, 5/1-6/04.

35. Shalev, A.Y., Friedman, M.J., Foa, E.B., & Keane, T.M. Integration and summary. In: Foa E.B., Keane, T.M., Friedman, M.J. (eds.) (2000). *Effective treatments for PTSD: Practice guidelines from the International Society for Traumatic Stress Studies* (pp. 359-379). New York: Guilford. 2000.

36. Kofoed, L., Friedman, M.J., & Peck, R. (1993). Alcoholism and drug abuse in patients with PTSD. *Psychiatric Quarterly, 64,* 151-171.

37. Koerner, K., & Linehan, M.M. (2000). Research on dialectical behavior therapy for patients with borderline personality disorder. *Psychiatr Clin North Am, 23,* 151-167.

38. Kinzie, D. (1989). Therapeutic approaches to traumatized Cambodian refugees. *Journal of Traumatic Stress, 2,* 75-91.

39. Gusman, F.D., Stewart, J., Young, B.H., Riney, S.J., Abueg, F.R. & Blake, D.D. (1996). A multicultural developmental approach for treating trauma. In A.J. Marsella, M.J. Friedman, E.T. Gerrity, & R.M. Scurfield (Eds.), *Ethnocultural aspects of posttraumatic stress disorder: Issues, research, and clinical applications* (pp. 439-458). Washington, DC, American Psychological Association.

40. Stamm, B.H. & Friedman, M.J. (1999). Transcultural perspectives on post-traumatic stress disorder and other reactions to extreme stress. In A. Shalev, R. Yehuda, & A. McFarlane (Eds.) *Human response to trauma across cultural, gender, and life course.* (pp. 69-85). New York, Plenum Press.

41. Marsella, A.J., Friedman, M.J., Gerrety, E.T. Scurfield, R.M. (1996). *Ethnocultural aspects of post-traumatic stress disorder: Issues, research and clinical applications.* Washington, DC, American Psychological Association

42. Roth, S. & Friedman, M.J. (Eds.) (1998). *Childhood trauma remembered: A report on the current scientific knowledge base and its applications.* Northbrook, IL, International Society for Traumatic Stress Studies.

43. Williams, L.M. (1994). Recall of childhood trauma: A prospective study of women's memories of child sexual abuse. *Journal of Consulting and Clinical Psychology, 62,* 1167-1176.

44. Herman, J.L., & Schatzow, E. (1987). Recovery and verification of memories of childhood sexual trauma. *Psychoanal Psychol, 4,* 1-14.

45. Schacter, D.L. (1996). *Search for memory.* New York: Basic Books.

46. Lindsay, D.S., Read, J.D. (1994). Psychotherapy and memories of childhood sexual abuse: A cognitive perspective. *Applied Cognitive Psychology, 8,* 281-338.

47. Brewin, C.R. (2003). *Posttraumatic Stress Disorder: Malady or Myth?* New Haven: Yale University Press.

48. Pope, K.S. (1996). Memory, abuse, and science: Questioning claims about the false memory syndrome epidemic. *American Psychologist, 51,* 957-974.

49. Schooler, J.W., Bendiksen, M., & Ambadar, Z. (1997). Taking the middle line: Can we accommodate both fabricated and recovered memories of sexual abuse? In I.M. Conway (Ed.), *False and recovered memories* (pp. 251-292). Oxford, Oxford University Press.

50. Loftus, E.F. (1993). The reality of repressed memories. *Amer Psychol, 48,* 518-537.

51. Loftus, E.F., Polonsky, S., Fullilove, M.T. (1994). Memories of childhood sexual abuse: Remembering and repressing. *Psychology of Women Quarterly, 18,* 67-84.

52. Elliott, D.M., & Briere, J. (1995). Posttraumatic stress associated with delayed recall of sexual abuse: A general population study. *Journal of Traumatic Stress, 8,* 629-648.

53. Chu, J.A. Frey, L.M., Ganzel, B.L., & Mathews, J.A. (1999). Memories of childhood abuse: Dissociation, amnesia, and corroboration. *American Journal of Psychiatry, 156,* 749-755.

54. Herman, J. (1992). *Trauma and recovery.* New York, Basic Books.

55. McCann, L., & Pearlman, A. (1990). Vicarious traumatization: A framework for understanding the psychological effects of working with victims. *Journal of Traumatic Stress, 3,* 131-149.

56. Figley, C.R. (1995). *Compassion fatigue: Secondary traumatic stress disorders from treating the traumatized.* New York, Brunner/Mazel.

57. Danieli, Y. (1984). Psychotherapists' participation in the conspiracy of silence about the Holocaust. *Psychoanalytic Psychology, 1,* 23-42.

58. Wilson, J. & Lindy, J. (1994). *Countertransference in the treatment of PTSD.* New York, Guilford Press.

59. Courtois, C.A. (1988). *Healing the incest wound: Adult survivors in therapy.* New York: WW Norton

60. Yassen, J. (1993). Group work with clinicians who have a history of trauma. *NCP Clinical Newsletter, 3:*10-11.

61. Rothbaum, B.O., Meadows, E.A., Resick, P., & Foy, D.W. (2000). Cognitive-behavioral treatment. In E.B. Foa, T.M. Keane, M.J. Friedman (Eds.), *Practice Guidelines for PTSD* (pp. 60-83). New York, Guilford.

62. Foa, E.B., & Kozak, M.J. (1986). Emotional processing of fear: Exposure to corrective information. *Psychological Bulletin, 99,* 20-35.

63. Foa, E.B., Riggs, D.S., Massie, E.G., & Yarczower, M. (1995). The impact of fear activation and anger on the efficacy of exposure treatment for PTSD. *Behavior Therapy, 26,* 487-499.

64. Follette, V.M., Ruzek, J.I., & Abueg, F.R. (1998). *Cognitive-behaviorlal therapies for trauma.* New York: Guildord.

65. Tarrier, N., Pilgrim, H., Sommerfield, C., et al. (1999). A randomized trial of cognitive therapy and imaginal exposure in the treatment of chronic posttraumatic stress disorder. *J Consult and Clin Psychol, 67,* 13-18.

66. Rothbaum, B.O., Hodges, L.F., Ready, D.J., Graap, K., & Alarcon, R.D. (2001). Virtual reality exposure therapy for Vietnam veterans with posttraumatic stress disorder. *Journal of Clinical Psychiatry, 62,* 617-622.

67. Lovell, K., Marks, I.M., Noshivarni, H., et al. (2001). Do cognitive and exposure treatments improve various PTSD symptoms differently? A randomized controlled trial. *Behav and Cognitive Psychotherapy, 29,* 107-112.

68. Resick, P., Nishith, P., Weaver, T., et al. (2002). A comparison of Cognitive Processing Therapy with Prolonged Exposure and a waiting condition for the treatment of chronic posttraumatic stress disorder in female rape victims. *J Consult and Clin Psychol, 70*, 867-879.

69. Hickling, E.J., & Blanchard, E.B. (1997). The private practice psychologist and manual-based treatments: Post-traumatic stress disorder secondary to motor vehicle accidents. *Behav Res Ther, 35*, 191-203.

70. Beck, A.T. (1976). *Cognitive therapy and the emotional disorders*. New York: International University Press.

71. Clark, D.M. (1986). A cognitive approach to panic. *Behaviour Research and Therapy, 24*, 461-470.

72. Marks, I., Lovell, K., Noshirvani, H., Livanou, M., & Thrasher, S. (1998). Treatment of post-traumatic stress disorder by exposure and/or cognitive restructuring: A controlled study. *Archives of General Psychiatry, 55*, 317-325.

73. Paunovic, N., & Ost, L. (2001). Cognitive-behavioral therapy vs. exposure therapy in the treatment of PTSD in refugees. *Behaviour Research and Therapy, 39*, 1183-1197.

74. Resick, P.A., & Schnicke, M.K. (1992). Cognitive processing therapy for sexual assault victims. *Journal of Consulting and Clinical Psychology, 60*, 748-756.

75. Resick, P.A., & Schnicke, M.K. (1993). *Cognitive processing therapy for rape victims: A treatment manual.* Newbury Park: SAGE Publications.

76. Kilpatrick, D.G., Veronen, L.J., & Resick, P.A. (1982). Psychological sequelae to rape: Assessment and treatment strategies. In D.M. Dolays & R.L. Meredith (Eds.), *Behavioral medicine: Assessment and treatment strategies*, pp. 473-497. New York, Plenum.

77. Resick, P.A., Jordan, C.G., Girelli, S.A., Hutter, C.K., & Marhoefer-Dvorak, S. (1988). A comparative victim study of behavioral group therapy for sexual assault victims. *Behavior Therapy, 19*, 385-401.

78. Foa E.B., Dancu, C.V., Hembree, E.A., et al. (1999). A comparison of exposure therapy, stress inoculation training, and their combination for reducing posttraumatic stress disorder in female assault victims. *J Consult and Clin Psychology, 67*, 194-200.

79. Foa, E.B., Rothbaum, B.O., Riggs, D.S., et al. (1991). Treatment of posttraumatic stress disorder in rape victims: A comparison between cognitive-behavioral procedures and counseling. *J Consulting and Clin Psychology, 59*, 715-723.

80. Lange, A., van de Ven, J.P., Schrieken, B., & Emmelkamp, P.M.G. (2001). INTERAPY: Treatment of post-traumatic stress through the Internet. *Journal of Behavior Therapy & Experimental Psychiatry, 32*, 73-90.

81. Lange, A., Rietdijk, D., Judcovicova, M., van de ven, J.P., Schrieken, B., & Emmelkamp, P.M.G. (2003). Interapy: A controlled randomized trial of the standard treatment of posttraumatic stress through the Internet. *Journal of Consulting & Clinical Psychology, 71*, 901-909.

82. Krakow, B., Hollifield, M., Johnston, L., et al. (2001). Imagery rehearsal therapy for chronic nightmares in sexual assault survivors with posttraumatic stress disorder: A randomized controlled trial. *Journal of the American Medical Association, 286*, 537-545.

83. Forbes, D., Phleps, A., & McHugh, T. (2001). Treatment of combat-related nightmares using imagery rehearsal: A pilot study. *J Trauma Stress, 14*, 433-442.

84. Krakow, B., Sandoval, D., Schrader, R., et al. (2001). Treatment of chronic nightmares in adjudicated adolescent girls in a residential facility. *J Adolesc Health, 29*, 94-100.

85. Evans, K., Tyrer, P., et al. (1999). Manual-assisted cognitive-behaviour therapy (MACT): A randomized controlled trial of a brief intervention with bibliotherapy in the treatment of recurrent deliberate self-harm. *Psychol Med, 29*, 19-25.

86. Hawton, K., Townsend, E., et al. (2000). *Psychosocial versus pharmacological treatments for deliberate self-harm.* Cochrane Database Syst Rev. CD001764.

87. Becker, C.B., & Zayfert, C. (2001). Integrating DBT-based techniques and concepts to facilitate exposure treatment for PTSD. *Cognitive & Behavioral Practice, 8*, 107-122.

88. Shapiro, F. (1989). Eye movement desensitization: A new treatment for post-traumatic stress disorder. *Journal of Behavior Therapy and Experimental Psychiatry, 20*, 211-217.

89. Shapiro, F. (1995). *Eye movement desensitization and reprocessing: Basic principles, protocols, and procedures.* New York, Guilford.

90. McNally, R.J. (1999). Research on eye movement desensitization and reprocessing (EMDR) as a treatment for PTSD. *PTSD Research Quarterly, 10,* 1-7.

91. Chemtob, C.M., Tolin, D.F., & van der Kolk, B.A. (2000). Guidelines for treatment of PTSD: Eye movement desensitization and reprocessing. *J Trauma Stress, 13,* 569-570.

92. Hyer, L. & Brandsma, J.M. (1997). EMDR minus eye movements equals good psychotherapy. *Journal of Traumatic Stress, 10,* 515-522.

93. Ironson, G., Freund, B., Strauss, J.L., et al. (2002). Comparison of two treatments for traumatic stress: A community-based study of EMDR and prolonged exposure. *J Clin Psychol, 58,* 113-128.

94. Jensen, J.A. (1994). An investigation of Eye Movement Desensitization and Reprocessing (EMD/R) as a treatment for Posttraumatic Stress Disorder (PTSD) symptoms of Vietnam combat veterans. *Behav Therapy, 25,* 311-325.

95. Devilly, G.J., & Spence, S.H. (1999). The relative efficacy and treatment distress of EMDR and a cognitive behavioral trauma treatment protocol in the amelioration of post traumatic stress disorder. *Journal of Anxiety Disorders, 13,* 131-158.

96. Foa, E., & Meadows, E. (1997). Psychosocial treatments for posttraumatic stress disorder: A critical review. *Ann Rev Psychol, 48,* 449-480.

97. Davidson, P.R., & Parker, K.C. (2001). Eye movement desensitization and reprocessing (EMDR): A meta-analysis. *J Consult & Clin Psychol, 69,* 305-316.

98. Maxfield, L., & Hyer, L. (2002). The relationship between efficacy and methodology in studies investigating EMDR treatment of PTSD. *J Clin Psychol, 58,* 23-41.

99. Shephard, J., Stein, K., & Milne, R. (2000). Eye movement desensitization and reprocessing in the treatment of post-traumatic stress disorder: A review of an emerging therapy. *Psychol Med, 30,* 863-871.

100. Kudler, H., Blank, A., Krupnick, J. (2000). The psychoanalytic psychotherapy of posttraumatic stress disorder. In E.B. Foa, T.M. Keane, & M.J. Friedman (Eds.), *Practice Guidelines for PTSD* (pp. 176-198). New York, Guilford.

101. Horowitz, M.J. (1974). Stress response syndromes: Character style and dynamic psychotherapy. *Archives of General Psychiatry, 31,* 768-781.

102. Krystal, H. (1988). *Integration and self healing.* Hillsdale, NJ, The Analytic Press.

103. Lindy, J. (1996). Psychoanalytic psychotherapy of post-traumatic stress disorder. In B. van der Kolk, A. McFarlane, & L. Weisaeth (Eds.), *Traumatic stress* (pp. 525-536). New York, Guilford Press.

104. Marmar, C. & Freeman, M. (1988). Brief dynamic psychotherapy for post-traumatic stress disorders: Management of narcissistic regression. *Journal of Traumatic Stress, 1,* 323-337.

105. Brom, D., Kleber, R.J., & Defares, P.B. (1989). Brief psychotherapy for post-traumatic stress disorders. *Journal of Consulting and Clinical Psychology, 57,* 607-612.

106. Foy, D.W., Glynn, S.M., Schnurr, P.P. Weiss, D.S. Wattenberg, M.S., Marmar, C.R., Kankowski, M.K., & Gusman, F.D. (2003). Group psychotherapy for posttraumatic stress disorder. In E.B. Foa, T.M. Keane, & M.J. Friedman (Eds.), *Practice Guidelines for PTSD.* New York, Guilford.

107. Yalom, I.D. (1975). The theory and practice of group psychotherapy. New York, Basic Books.

108. Roth, S.H., Dye, E., & Lebowitz, L. (1988). Group therapy for sexual assault victims. *Psychotherapy, 25,* 82-93.

109. Foy, D.W., Glynn, S.M., Schnurr, P.P., Weiss, D.S., Wattenberg, M.S., Marmar, C.R., Kankowski, M.K. & Gusman, F.D. (2000). Group psychotherapy for posttraumatic stress disorder. In E.B. Foa, T.M. Keane & M.J. Friedman (Eds.), *Effective Treatmenst for PTSD: Practice Guidelines from the International Society for Traumatic Stress Studies* (pp. 153-175). New York: Guilford.

110. Foy, D.W., Ruzek, J.I., Glynn, S.M., Riney, S.A., & Gusman, F.D. (1997). Trauma focus group therapy for combat-related PTSD. *In Session: Psychotherapy in Practice, 3,* 59-73.

111. Rogers, S.S. & Silver, M., et al. (1999). A single session group study of exposure and Eye Movement Desensitization and Reprocessing in treating Posttraumatic Stress Disorder among Vietnam War veterans: Preliminary data. *J Anxiety Disord, 13,* 119-130.

112. Schnurr, P.P., Friedman, M.J., Foy, D.W., Shea, M.T., Hsieh, F.Y., Lavori, P.W., Glynn, S.M., Wattenberg, M.S., Bernardy, N.C. (2003). Randomized trial of trauma-focused group therapy for posttraumatic stress disorder. *Archives of General Psychiatry, 60*, 481-489.

113. Riggs, D.S. (2000). Marital and family therapy. In E.B. Foa, T.M. Keane, M.J. Friedman (Eds.), *Practice Guidelines for PTSD* (pp. 280-301). New York, Guilford.

114. Waysman, M., Mikulincer, M., Solomon, Z., et al. (1993). Secondary traumatization among wives of post-traumatic combat veterans: A family typology. *Journal of Family Psychology, 7*, 104-118.

115. Figley, C.R. (1989). *Helping traumatized families*. San Francisco, Jossey-Bass.

116. Johnson, D.R., Feldman, S.C., & Lubin, H. (1995). Critical interaction therapy: Couples therapy in combat-related posttraumatic stress disorder. *Family Process, 34*, 401-412.

117. Harris, C.J. (1991). A family crisis-intervention model for the treatment of post-traumatic stress reaction. *Journal of Traumatic Stress, 4*, 195-207.

118. Rosenheck, R. & Thompson, J. (1986). "Detoxification" of Vietnam war trauma: A combined family-individual approach. *Family Process, 25*, 559-570.

119. Williams, C.M. & Williams, T. (1980). Family therapy for Vietnam veterans. In T. Williams (Ed.), *Post-traumatic stress disorder of the Vietnam veteran*. Cincinnati, OH, Disabled American Veterans.

120. Cardena, E., Maldonado, J., van der Hart, O., & Spiegel, D. (2000). Hypnosis. In E.B. Foa, T.M. Keane, & M.J. Friedman (Eds.), *Practice Guidelines for PTSD* (pp. 247-279. New York: Guilford.

121. Mueser, K.T., Salyers, M.P., Rosenberg, S.D., Ford, J.D., Fox, L., & Carty, P. (2001). Psychometric evaluation of trauma and posttraumatic stress disorder assessments in persons with severe mental illness. *Psychological Assessment, 13*, 110-117.

122. Penk, W. Binus, G., Herz, L. et al. (2000). Psychosocial rehabilitation techniques. In E.B. Foa, T.M. Keane, & M.J. Friedman (Eds.), *Practice Guidelines for PTSD*, (pp 224-246). New York, Guilford.

123. Pynoos, R.S. (1993). Traumatic stress and developmental psychopathology in children and adolescents. In *Review of Psychiatry, Volume 12* (pp. 205-238). J.M. Oldham, M.B. Riba, & A. Tasman (Eds.), Washington, DC: American Psychiatric Press, Inc.

124. Pynoos, R.S., Steinberg, A.M., Wraith, R. (1995). A developmental model of childhood traumatic stress. In D. Cicchetti, & D. Cohen (Eds.), *Manual of developmental psychology, vol 2: Risk, disorder, and adaptation*. New York, John Wiley.

125. Terr, L.C. (1989). Treating psychic trauma in children. *Journal of Traumatic Stress, 2*, 3-19.

126. Putnam, F.W. (1997). *Dissociation in children and adolescents: A developmental perspective*. New York, Guilford.

127. Herman, J.L., Perry, J.C., van der Kolk, B.A. (1989). Childhood trauma in borderline personality disorder. *American Journal of Psychiatry, 146*, 490-495.

128. Lyons, J.A. (1987). Posttraumatic stress disorder in children and adolescents: A review of the literature. *Dev Behav Pediatr, 8*, 349-356.

129. Cohen, J.A., Mannarino, A.P. (1998). Interventions for sexually abused children: Initial treatment findings. *Child Maltreatment, 3*, 17-26.

130. Deblinger, E., Lippman, J., Steer, R. (1996). Sexually abused children suffering posttraumatic stress symptoms: Initial treatment outcome findings. *Child Maltreatment, 1*, 310-321.

131. Chemtob, C.M., Tomas, S., Law, W., Cremniter, D. (1997). Postdisaster psychosocial intervention: A field study of the impact of debriefing on psychological distress. *American Journal of Psychiatry, 154*, 415-417.

132. Goenjian, A.K., Pynoos, R.S., Steinberg, A.M. et al. (1995). Psychiatric comorbidity in children after the 1988 earthquake in Armenia. *Journal of the American Academy of Child & Adolescent Psychiatry, 34*, 1174-1184.

133. March, J.L., Amaya-Jackson, L. et al. (1998). Cognitive-behavioral psychotherapy for children and adolescents with post-traumatic stress disorder following a single incident stressor. *Journal of the American Academy of Child and Adolescent Psychiatry, 37*, 585-593.

134. Cohen, J.A., Berliner, L., & March, J.S. (2000). PTSD treatment guidelines for children and adolescents. In E.B. Foa, T.M. Keane, & M.J. Friedman (Eds.), *Practice Guidelines for PTSD*, (pp 106-108). New York, Guilford.

135. Cannon, W.B. (1932). *The Wisdom of the Body*. New York: Norton.

136. Selye, H. (1946). The general adaptation syndrome and the diseases of adaptation. *J Clin Endocrinol, 6*: 117-230.

137. Chrousos, G.P., Gold, P.W. (1992). The concepts of stress and stress system disorders: Overview of physical and behavioral homeostasis. *JAMA, 267*, 1244-1252.

138. Southwick, S.M., Paige, S.R., Morgan, C.A., Bremner, J.D., Krystal, J.H., Charney, D.S. (1999). Adrenergic and serotonergic abnormalities in PTSD: Catecholamines and serotonin. *Seminars in Clinical Neuropsychiatry, 4*, 242-248.

139. Malloy, P., Fairbank, J., Keane, T. (1983). Validation of a multimethod assessment of posttraumatic stress disorder in Vietnam veterans. *J Consult Clin Psychol, 51*, 488-493.

140. Pitman, R., Orr, S., Forgue, D., et al. (1987). Psychophysiologic assessment of posttraumatic stress disorder imagery in Vietnam combat veterans. *Arch Gen Psychiatry, 44*, 970-975.

141. Southwick, S.M., Krystal, J.H., Morgan, A.C., et al. (1993). Abnormal noradrenergic function in post-traumatic stress disorder. *Arch Gen Psychiatry, 50*, 266-274 .

142. Bremner, J.D., Licinio, J., Darnell, A., et al. (1997). Elevated CRF corticotropin-releasing factor concentrations in post-traumatic stress disorder. *Am J Psychiatry 154*, 624-629.

143. Yehuda R, McFarlane A.C. (1995). Conflict between current knowledge about posttraumatic stress disorder and its original conceptual basis. *Am J Psychiatry, 152*, 1705-1713.

144. Friedman, M.J., (2003). Pharmacological management of PTSD. *Primary Psychiatry, 10*, 66-73.

145. Friedman, M.J., Davidson, J.R.T., Mellman, T.A., & Southwick, S.M. (2000). Guidelines for pharmacotherapy and position paper on practice guidelines. In: Foa, E.B., Keane, T.M., Friedman, M.J., eds. *Effective Treatments for Post-traumatic Stress Disorder: Practice Guidelines from the International Society for Traumatic Stress Studies.* (pp. 84-105). New York, NY: Guilford.

146. Friedman, M.J., Donnelly, C.L., & Mellman, T.A. (2003). Pharmacotherapy for PTSD. *Psychiatric Annals, 22*, 57-62.

147. Brady, K. Pearlstein, T., & Asnis, G.M., et al. (2000). Efficacy and safety of sertraline treatment of posttraumatic stress disorder. *JAMA, 283*, 1837-1844.

148. Davidson, J.R.T., Rothbaum, B.O., & van der Kolk, B.A., et al. (2001). Multicenter, double-blind comparison of sertraline and placebo in the treatment of posttraumatic stress disorder. *Archives of General Psychiatry, 58*, 485-492.

149. Marshall, R.D., Beebe, K.L., Oldham, M., & Zaninelli, R. (2001). Efficacy and safety of paroxetine treatment for chronic PTSD: A fixed-dose-placebo-controlled study. *American Journal of Psychiatry, 158*, 1982-1988.

150. Tucker, P., Zaninelli, R., Yehuda, R., Ruggiero, L., Dillingham, K., & Pitts, C.D. (2001). Paroxetine in the treatment of chronic posttraumatic stress disorder: Results of a placebo-controlled, flexible-dosage trial. *Journal of Clinical Psychiatry, 62*, 860-868.

151. Martenyi, F., Brown, E.B., Zhang, H., Prakash, A., & Koke, S.C. (2002). Fluoxetine versus placebo in posttraumatic stress disorder. *Journal of Clinical Psychiatry, 63*, 199-206.

152. Seedat, S., Lockhat, R., Kaminer, D., Zungu-Dirwayi, N., & Stein, D.J. (2001). An open trial of citalopram in adolescents with post-traumatic stress disorder. *Int Clin Psychopharmacol, 16*, 21-25.

153. Lonborg, P.D., Hegel, M.T., Goldstein, S., Goldstein, D., Himmelhoch, J.M., Maddock, R., Patterson, W.M., Rausch, J., & Farfel, G.M. (2001). Sertraline treatment of posttraumatic stress disorder: Results of weeks of open-label continuation treatment. *J Clin Psychiatry, 62*, 325-331.

154. Whittington, C. J., Kendall, R., Fonagy, P., Cottrell, D., Cotgrove, A., and Boddington, E. (2004). Selective serotonin reuptake inhibitors in childhood depression: systematic review of published versus unpublished data. *The Lancet, 363*, 1341-45.

155. U.S. Food and Drug Administration (2004). *FDA Talk Paper: FDA Issues Public Health Advisory on Cautions for Use of Antidepressants in Adults and Children* (T04-08, March 22, 2004). Retrieved from: http://www.fda.gov.

156. Davidson, J.R.T., Lipschitz, A., Musgnung, J. (2004). Treatment of PTSD with venlafaxine XR, sertraline, or placebo; a doubleblind comparison, *Intl. J. Neuropsycho-pharmacology 7*, 1 P:02.228.

157. DeMartino, R., Mollica, R.F., Wilk, V. (1995). Monoamine oxidase inhibitors in posttraumatic stress disorder. *J Nerv Ment Dis 183*, 510-515.

158. Southwick, S.M., Yehuda, R., Giller, E.L. et al. (1994). Use of tricyclics and monoamine oxidase inhibitors in the treatment of PTSD: A quantitative review. Murburg MM (ed), pp 293-305. *Catecholamine function in post-traumatic stress disorder: Emerging concepts.* American Psychiatry Press, Washington, DC.

159. Raskind, M.A., Peskind, E.R., Kanter, E.D., Petrie, E.C., Radont, A., Thompson, C., Dobie, D.J., Hoff, D., Rein, R.J., Straits-Troster, K., Thomas R., & McFall, M.M. (2002). Prazosin reduces nightmares and other PTSD symptoms in combat veterans: A placebo-controlled study. *American Journal of Psychiatry 63*, 565-568.

160. Famularo, R., Kinscherff, R., & Fenton, T. (1988). Propranolol treatment for childhood posttraumatic stress disorder, acute type. *Am J Dis Child, 142*, 1244-1247.

161. Kinzie, J.D., & Friedman, M.J. (2004). Psychopharmacology for refugee and asylum seeker patients. In J. P. Wilson, B. Drozdek, eds. *Broken spirits: The treatment of asylum seekers and refugees with PTSD.* pp. 579-600, New York: Brunner-Routledge Press.

162. Post, R.M., Weiss, S.R.B., Smith, M.A. (1995). Sensitization and kindling: Implications for the evolving neural substrate of PTSD. Friedman, M.J., Charney, D.S., Deutch, A.Y., (eds), (pp 203-224). *Neurobiological and Clinical Consequences of Stress: From Normal Adaptation to PTSD.* Lippincott-Raven Press, Philadelphia, PA .

163. Friedman, M.J., Southwick, S.M. (1995). Towards pharmacotherapy for PTSD. Friedman, M.J., Charney, D.S., Deutch, A.Y. (eds), pp 465-481. *Neurobiological and Clinical Consequences of Stress: From Normal Adaptation to PTSD.* Lippincott-Raven Press, Philadelphia, PA.

164. Braun, P., Greenberg, D., Dasberg, H. et al. (1990). Core symptoms of posttraumatic stress disorder unimproved by alprazolam treatment. *J Clin Psychiatry 51*, 236-238.

165. Monnelly, E.P., Ciraulo, D.A., Knapp, C., & Keane, T. (1999). Low dose risperidone as adjunctive therapy for irritable aggression in posttraumatic stress disorder. *J Clinical Psychopharmacology, 19*, 377-378.

166. Norris, F., Friedman, M., Watson, P., Byrne, C., Diaz, E., & Kaniasty, K. (2002). 60,000 disaster victims speak, Par I: An empirical review of the empirical literature, 1981 – 2001. *Psychiatry, 65*, 207-239.

167. Norris, F., Friedman, M., & Watson, P. (2002). 60,000 disaster victims speak, Part II: Summary and implications of the disaster mental health research. *Psychiatry, 65*, 240-260.

168. Norris, F.H., Murphy, A.D., Baker, C.K., Perilla, J.L (2003). Severity, timing and duration of reactions to trauma in the population: An example from Mexico. *Biol Psychiatry, 53*, 769-778.

169. Schuster, M., Bradley, D., Stein, M., Jaycox, L.H., Collins, R.L., Marshall, G.N., Elliott, M.N., Zhou, A.J., Kanouse, D.E., Morrison, J.L., & Berry, S.H. (2001). A national survey of stress reactions after the September 11, 2001, terrorist attacks. *New England Journal of Medicine, 345*, 1507-1512.

170. Galea, S., Ahern, J., Resnick, H.S., Kilpatrick, D.G., Bucuvalas, M.J., Gold, J., & Vlahov, D. (2002). Psychological sequelae of the September 11 terrorist attacks in New York City. *New England Journal of Medicine, 346*, 982-987.

171. Daviss, W.B., Racusin, R., Fleischer, A., Mooney, D., Ford, J.D., McHugo, G.J. (2000). Acute stress disorder symptomatology during hospitalization for pediatric injury. *J Am Acad Child Adolesc Psychiatry 39*, 569-575.

172. Classen, C., Koopman, C., Hales, R., Spiegel, D. (1998). Acute stress disorder as a predictor of posttraumatic stress symptoms. *Am J Psychiatry, 155*: 620-624.

173. Eriksson, N.G., Lundin, T. (1996). Early traumatic stress reactions among Swedish survivors of the m/s Estonia disaster. *Br J Psychiatry, 169*: 713-716.

174. Staab, J.P., Grieger, T.A., Fullerton, C.S., Ursano, R.J. (1996). Acute stress disorder, subsequent posttraumatic stress disorder and depression after a series of typhoons. *Anxiety, 2*: 219-225.

175. Bryant, R.A., Harvey, A.G.. (1998). Relationship between acute stress disorder and posttraumatic stress disorder following mild traumatic brain injury. *Am J Psychiatry, 155*: 625-629.

176. Bryant, R.A. (2003). Early predictors of posttraumatic stress disorder. *Biological Psychiatry, 53*, 789-795.

177. Shalev, A.Y., Sahar, T., Freedman, S., Peri, T., Glick, N., Brandes, D., et al., (1998). A prospective study of heart rate response following trauma and subsequent development of posttraumatic stress disorder. *Arch Gen Psychiatry, 55*, 553-559.

178. Ehlers, A., Clark, D.M. (2003). Early psychological interventions for adult survivors of trauma: A review. *Biol Psychiatry, 53*, 817-826.

179. Watson, P.J., Shalev, A.Y. (2005). Assessment and treatment of adult acute responses to traumatic stress following mass traumatic events. *CNS Spectr., Feb; 10(2)*, 123-31.

180. Friedman, M.J. (2005). Towards a public mental health approach for survivors of bioterrorism. In Y. Danieli & D. Brom (Eds.), *The Trauma of Terror: Sharing Knowledge and Shared Care.* (pp. 527-540). New York: Guilford.

181. Naturale, A.J. (in press). Mental health outreach strategies: An experiential description of the outreach methodologies utilized in the New York 9/11 disaster response. In E.C. Ritchie, M.J. Friedman, & P.J. Watson (Eds.), *Psychological and public health interventions followi ng mass violence and disasters.* New York: Guilford Press.

182. Solomon, Z. & Benbenishty, R. (1986). The role of proximity, immediacy, and expectancy in frontline treatment of combat stress reaction among Israelis in the Lebanon War. *American Journal of Psychiatry, 143*, 613-617.

183. Mitchell, J.T. (1983). When disaster strikes...*Journal Of Emergency Medical Services, 8*, 36-39.

184. Dyregrov, A. (1989). Caring for helpers in disaster situations: Psychological debriefing. *Disaster Management, 2*, 25-30.

185. Bisson, J.I., McFarlane, A.C., & Rose, S. (2000). Psychological debriefing. In E.B. Foa, T.M. Keane, & M.J. Friedman (Eds.), *Practice Guidelines for PTSD* (pp. 39-59). New York, Guilford.

186. Rose, S., Bisson, J., Wessely, S. (2002). Psychological debriefing for preventing post traumatic stress disorder (PTSD) (Chochrane review). In: *The Cochrane Library, Issue 2 2002.* Oxford, UK: Update Software.

187. Bisson, J.I., Jenkins, P.L., Alexander, J., Bannister, C. (1997). Randomized controlled trial of psychological debriefing for victims of acute burn trauma. *Br J Psychiatry, 171*, 78-81.

188. Mayou, R.A., Ehlers, A., Hobbs, M. (2000). A three-year follow-up of psychological debriefing for road traffic accident victims. *Br J Psychiatry, 176*, 589-593.

189. Rauch, S.A.M., Hembree, E.A., Foa, E.B. (2001). Acute psychosocial preventive interventions for PTSD. *Advances In Mind-Body Medicine, 17*, 187-191.

190. Ehlers, A., Steil, R. (1995). *An experimental study of intrusive memories.* Paper presented at the World Congress of Behavioural and Cognitive Therapies; Copenhagen, Denmark.

191. Foa, E.B., Cahill, S.P. (2001). Psychological therapies: Emotional processing. In NJ Smelser, PBBates (Eds.) *International Encyclopedia of the Social and Behavioral Sciences.* Oxford:Elsvier (pp. 12363-12369).

192. Bryant, R.A. (2003). Early predictors of posttraumatic stress disorder. *Biol Psychiatry, 53*, 789-795.

193. McNally, R J. (2003). Psychological mechanisms in acute response to trauma. *Biol Psychiatry, 53*, 779-788.

194. Bryant, R.A., Harvey, A.G., Guthrie, R.M., Moulds, M.L. (2000). A prospective study of psychophysiological arousal, acute stress disorder and posttraumatic stress disorder. *J Abnorm Psychol, 109*, 341-344.

195. Morgan, C.A., Krystal, J.H., Southwick, S.M. (2003). Toward early pharmacologic post-traumatic stress intervention. *Biol Psychiatry, 53*, 834-843.

196. Bryant RA, Harvey AG, Dang ST, et al. (1998). Treatment of acute stress disorder: A comparison of cognitive-behavioral therapy and supportive counseling. *J Consult Clin Psychol, 66*, 862-866.

197. Bryant RA, Sackville T, Dang ST, et al. (1999). Treating acute stress disorder: An evaluation of cognitive behavior therapy and supportive counseling techniques. *Am J Psychiatry, 156*, 1780-1786.

198. Bryant, RA, Moulds, M.L., Nixon, R.D.V. (2003). Cognitive therapy of acute stress disorder: A four-year follow-up. *Behav Res Ther, 41*, 489-494.

199. Foa, E.B., Hearst-Ikeda, D., Perry, K.J. (1995). Evaluation of a brief cognitive-behavioral program for the prevention of chronic PTSD in recent assault victims. *J Consult Clin Psychol, 63*, 948-955.

200. Cohen, J.A. (2003). Treating acute posttraumatic reactions in children and adolescents. *Biol Psychiatry, 53*, 827-833.

201. Robert, R, Blakeney, P.E., Villarreal, C., Rosenberg, L., Meyer, W.J. 3rd (1999). Imipramine treatment in pediatric burn patients with symptoms of acute stress disorder: a pilot study. *J Am Acad Child Adolesc Psychiatry, 38*, 873-882.

202. Saxe, G., Stoddar, F., Courtney, D., Cunningham, K., Chawla, N., Sheridan, R., King, D., King, L. (2001). Relationship between acute morphine and the course of PTSD in children with burns. *J Am Child Adolesc Psychiatry, 40*, 915-921.

203. Pitman, R., Sanders, K.M., Zusman, R.M., Healy, A.R., Cheema. F., Lasko, N.B. et al. (2002). Pilot study of secondary prevention of posttraumatic stress disorder with propranolol. *Biol Psychiatry, 51*, 189-192.

204. Taylor, F., Cahill, L. (2002). Propranolol for reemergent posttraumatic stress disorder following an event of retraumatization: A case study. *J Traumatic Stress, 15*, 433-437.

205. Guillaume, V., Francois, D., Karine, J., Benoit, A., Philippe, L., Alain, B., Marmar, C. (in press). Immediate treatment with propranolol decreases PTSD two months after trauma. *Biol Psychiatry.*

206. Norris, F., & Hamblen, J. (2004). Standardized self-report measures of civilian trauma and PTSD. In J.P. Wilson & T.M. Keane (Eds.), *Assessing psychological trauma and PTSD, Second Edition.* pp 63-102, New York: Guilford Publications.

207. Norris, F. (1992). Epidemiology of trauma: Frequency and impact of different potentially traumatic events on different demographic groups. *Journal of Consulting and Clinical Psychology, 60*, 409-418.

208. Kilpatrick, D., Resnick, H., & Freedy, J. (1991). *The Potential Stressful Events Interview.* Unpublished instrument, Medical University of South Carolina, Charleston, South Carolina.

209. Vrana, S., & Lauterbach, D. (1994). Prevalence of traumatic events and post-traumatic psychological symptoms in a nonclinical sample of college students. *Journal of Traumatic Stress, 7*, 289-302.

210. Krinsley, K.E., & Weathers, F.W. (1995). The assessment of trauma in adults. *PTSD Research Quarterly, 6*, 1-6.

211. Green, B.L. (1996). Trauma History Questionnaire. In B.H. Stamm & E.M. Varra (Eds.), *Measurement of stress, trauma, and adaptation* (pp. 366-368). Lutherville, MD: Sidran Press.

212. Kubany, E., Haynes, S., Leisen, M., Owens, J., Kaplan, A., Watson, S., & Burns, K. (2000). Development and preliminary validation of a brief broad-spectrum measure of trauma exposure: The Traumatic Life Events Questionnaire. *Psychological Assessment, 12*, 210-224.

213. Goodman, L., Corcoran, C., Turner, K., Yuan, N., & Green, B. (1998). Assessing traumatic event exposure: General issues and preliminary findings for the Stressful Life Events Screening Questionnaire. *Journal of Traumatic Stress, 11*, 521-542.

214. Wolfe, J., Kimerling, R., Brown, P.J., Chrestman, K.R., & Levin, K. (1996). Psychometric review of the Life Stressor Checklist-Revised. In B.H. Stamm & E.M. Varra (Eds.), *Measurement of stress, trauma, and adaptation.* Lutherville, MD: Sidran Press (pp. 198-201).

215. Sanders, B., & Becker-Lausen, E. (1995). The measurement of psychological maltreatment: Early data on the Child Abuse and Trauma Scale. *Child Abuse & Neglect, 19*, 315-323.

216. Bernstein, D.P., Fink, L., Handelsman, L. et al. (1994). Initial reliability and validity of a new retrospective measure of child abuse and neglect. *American Journal of Psychiatry, 151*, 1132-1136.

217. Ogata, S.N., Silk, K.R., Goodrich, S., Lohr, N.E., Westen, D., & Hill, E.M (1990). Childhood sexual and physical abuse in adult patients with borderline personality disorder. *American Journal of Psychiatry, 147*, 1008-1013.

218. Gallagher, R.E., Flye, B.L., Hurt, S.W., Stone, M.H., & Hull, J.W. (1992). Retrospective assessment of traumatic experiences (RATE). *Journal of Personality Disorders, 6*, 99-108.

219. Bremner, J.D., Randall, P., Scott, T.M., Capelli, S., Delany, R., McCarthy, G., Charney, D.S. (1995). Deficits in short-term memory in adult survivors of childhood abuse. *Psychiatry Research, 59*, 97-107.

220. Straus, M. (1979). Measuring intrafamily conflict and violence: The Conflict Tactics (CT) Scales. *Journal of Marriage and the Family, 41*, 75-88.

221. Shepard, M.F., & Campbell, J.A. (1992). The Abusive Behavior Inventory: A measure of psychological and physical abuse. *Journal of Interpersonal Violence, 7*, 291-305.

222. Koss, M.P., & Gidycz, C.A. (1985). Sexual experiences survey: Reliability and validity. *Journal of Consulting and Clinical Psychology, 53*, 422-423.

223. Wyatt, G.E., Lawrence, J., Vodounon, A., & Mickey, M.R. (1992). The Wyatt Sex History Questionnaire: A structured interview for female sexual history taking. *Journal of Child Sexual Abuse, 1(4)*, 51-68.

224. Keane, T.M., Fairbank, J.A., Caddell, J.M., Zimering, R.T., Taylor, K.L., & Mora, C.A. (1989). Clinical evaluation of a measure to assess combat exposure. *Psychological Assessment, 1*, 53-55.

225. Wolfe, J., Brown, P.J., Furey, J., & Levin, K.B. (1993). Development of a wartime stressor scale for women. *Psychological Assessment, 5*, 330-335.

226. Mollica, R.F., Caspi-Yavin, Y., Bollini, P., Truong, T., Tor, S., & Lavelle, J. (1992). The Harvard Trauma Questionnaire: Validating a cross-cultural instrument for measuring torture, trauma, and posttraumatic stress disorder in Indochinese refugees. *Journal of Nervous and Mental Disease, 180*, 111-116.

227. First MB, Spitzer, R.L., Williams, J.B.W., & Gibbon, M (1996). *Structured Clinical Interview for DSM-IV*. New York: New York State Psychiatric Institute, Biometrics Research.

228. Blake, D.D., Weathers, F.W., Nagy, L.M., Kaloupek, D.G., Gusman, F.D., Charney, D.S., & Keane, T.M. (1995). The development of a clinician-administered PTSD scale. *Journal of Traumatic Stress, 8*, 75-90.

229. Watson, C., Juba, M., Manifold, V., Kucala, T., & Anderson, P. (1991). The PTSD Interview: Rationale, description, reliability and concurrent validity of a DSM-III based technique. *Journal of Clinical Psychology, 47*, 179-185.

230. Davidson, J.R.T., Book, S.W., Colket, J.T., Tupler, L.A., Roth, S., David, D., Hertzberg, M., Mellman, T., Beckham, J.C., Smith, R.D., Davidson, R.M., Katz, R & Feldman, M.E. (1997). Assessment of a new self-rating scale for posttraumatic stress disorder. *Psychological Medicine, 27*, 153-160.

231. World Health Organization (1997). *Composite International Diagnostic Interview (CIDI)*, Version 2.1. Geneva: World Health Organization.

232. Foa, E., Cashman, L., Jaycox, L., & Perry, K. (1997). The validation of a self-report measure of posttraumatic stress disorder. *Psychological Assessment, 9*, 445-451.

233. Robins, L.M., Cottler, L., Bucholz, K. (1995). *Diagnostic Interview Schedule for DSM-IV*. St Louis: Washington University

234. Breslau, N., Kessler, R., Peterson, E.L. (1998). PTSD assessment with a structured interview: Reliability and concordance with a standard clinical interview. *International Journal of Methods & Psychiatric Research, 7*, 121-127.

235. Weathers, F.W., Litz, B.T., Herman, D.S., Huska, J.A. & Keane, T.M. (1995). *PTSD Checklist (PCL)*. Boston, National Center for PTSD.

236. Foa, E., Riggs, D., Dancu, C., & Rothbaum, B. (1993). Reliability and validity of a brief instrument for assessing post-traumatic stress disorder. *Journal of Traumatic Stress, 6*, 459-474.

237. Lyons, J., & Keane, T. (1992). Keane PTSD Scale: MMPI and MMPI-2 update. *Journal of Traumatic Stress, 5*, 111-117.

238. Schlenger, W., & Kulka, R.A. (1989). *PTSD scale development for the MMPI-2*. Research Triangle Park, NC: Research Triangle Park Institute.

239. Saunders, B., Arata, C., & Kilpatrick, D. (1990). Development of a crime-related posttraumatic stress disorder scale for women with the Symptom Checklist-90 Revised. *Journal of Traumatic Stress, 3*, 439-448.

240. Ursano, R., Fullerton, C., Kao, T., Bhartiya, V. (1995). Longitudinal assessment of posttraumatic stress disorder and depression following exposure to traumatic death. *Journal of Nervous and Mental Disease, 183*, 36-42.

241. Weiss, D.S., & Marmar, C.R. (1997). The Impact of Event Scale —Revised. In J.P. Wilson & T.M. Keane (Eds.), *Assessing psychological trauma and PTSD* (pp. 399-411). Guilford Press: London.

242. Keane, T.M., Caddell, J.M., & Taylor, K.L. (1988). Mississippi Scale for Combat-Related Posttraumatic Stress Disorder: Three studies in reliability and validity. *Journal of Consulting and Clinical Psychology, 56*, 85-90.

243. Norris, F., & Perilla, J. (1996). Reliability, validity, and cross-language stability of the Revised Civilian Mississippi Scale for PTSD. *Journal of Traumatic Stress, 9*, 285-298.

244. Hammarberg, M. (1992). Penn Inventory for Posttraumatic Stress Disorder: Psychometric properties. *Psychological Assessment, 4*, 67-76.

245. Briere, J., & Runtz, M. (1989). The Trauma Symptom Checklist (TSC-33): Early data on a new scale. *Journal of Interpersonal Violence, 4*, 151-163.

246. Briere, J. (1995). *Trauma Symptom Inventory (TSI): Professional manual*. Odessa, FL: Psychological Assessment Resources.

247. Nader, K.O. (1997). Assessing Traumatic Experiences in Children. In J.P. Wilson & T.M. Keane (Eds.), *Assessing psychological trauma and PTSD* (pp. 291-). Guilford Press: London.

248. National Center for Study of Corporal Punishment and Alternatives in Schools. (1992). *My Worst Experience Survey*. Philadelphia, PA: Temple University Press.

249. Ribbe, D. (1996). Psychometric review of Traumatic Event Screening Instrument for Children (TESI-C). In Stamm, B.H. (Ed.). (1996). *Measurement of stress, trauma and adaptation* (pp. 386-387). Lutherville, MD: Sidran Press.

250. Fletcher, K. (1991). *When Bad Things Happen Scale*. (Available from the author, University of Massachusetts Medical Center, Dept. of Psychiatry, 55 Lake Avenue North, Worcester, MA 01655.)

251. Friedrich, W. (1995). Evaluation and treatment: The clinical use of the Child Sexual Behavior Inventory: Commonly asked questions. *American Professional Society on the Abuse of Children (APSAC) Advisor, 8(1)*, 17-20.

252. Praver, F. (1994). *Child Rating Scales - Exposure to Interpersonal Abuse*. Unpublished copyrighted instrument.

253. Praver, F., Pelcovitz, D., & DiGiuseppe, R. (1994). *The Angie/Andy Child Rating Scales*, (Available from Praver, 5 Marseilles Drive, Locust Valley, NY 11560; Pelcovitz, Dept. of Psychiatry, 400 Community Drive, Manhasset, NY 11030; or DiGiuseppe, Psychology Dept. St. John's University, Grand Central and Utopia Parkways, Jamaica, NY 11439.)

254. Reich, W., Shayka, J.J., & Taibleson, C. (1991). *Diagnostic Interview for Children and Adolescents (DICA)*. St. Louis, MO: Washington University.

255. Nader, K.O., Kriegler, J.A., Blake, D.D., & Pynoos, R.S. (1994b). *Clinician Administered PTSD Scale, Child and Adolescent Version (CAPS-C)*. White River Junction, VT: National Center for PTSD.

256. Shaffer, D., Fisher, P., Dulcan, M., Davies, M., Piacentini, J., Schwab-Stone, M., Lahey, B.B., Bourdon, K., Jensen, P., Bird, H., Canino, G., & Regier, D. (in press). The NIMH Diagnostic Interview Schedule for Children (DISC-2.3): Description, acceptability, prevalences, and performance in the MECA study. *Journal of the American Academy of Child and Adolescent Psychiatry*.

257. Ohan, J., Myers, K., & Collett, B. (2002). Ten-year review of rating scales IV: Scales assessing trauma and its effects. *Journal of the American Academy of Child and Adolescent Psychiatry, 41*, 1401-1422.

258. Saigh, P.A., Yasik, A.E., Oberfield, R.A., Green, B.L., Halamandaris, P.V., Rubenstein, H., Nester, J., Resko, J., Hetz, B., & McHugh, M. (2000). The Children's PTSD Inventory: development and reliability. *Journal of Traumatic Stress, 13*, 369-380.

259. Yasik, A., Saigh, P., Oberfield, R., Green, B., Halamandaris, P. McHugh, M. (2001). The validity of the Children's PTSD Inventory. *Journal of Traumatic Stress, 14*, 81-94.

260. Steinberg, A.M., Brymer, M.J., Decker, K.B., Pynoos, R.S. (2004). The University of California at Los Angeles Post-Traumatic Stress Disorder Reaction Index. *Current Psychiatry Reports, 6*, 96-100.

261. Jones, R.T. (1994). *Child's Reaction to Traumatic Events Scale (CRTES): A self report traumatic stress measure*. (Available from the author, Dept. of Psychology, Stress and coping Lab, 4102 Derring Hall, Virginia Polytechnic Institute and State University, Blacksburg, VA 24060)

262. Wolfe, V.V., Wolfe, D.A., Gentile, C., & Larose, L. (1986). *Children's Impact of Traumatic Events Scale (CITES)*. (Available from Wolfe, Dept. of Psychology, London Health Sciences Center, 800 Commissioners Road East, London, Ontario (N6A4G5)

263. Chaffin, M., & Shultz, S.K. (2001). Psychometric evaluation of the Children's Impact of Traumatic Events Scale-Revised. *Child Abuse and Neglect, 25*, 401-411.

264. Briere, J. (1996a). *Trauma Symptom Checklist for Children (TSCC)*. Odessa, FL: Psychological Assessment Resources.

265. Briere, J. (1996b). *Trauma Symptom Checklist for Children (TSCC) professional manual*. Odessa, FL: Psychological Assessment Resources.

266. Foa, E.B., Johnson, K.M., Feeny, N.C., & Treadwell, K.R. (2001). The Child PTSD Symptom Scale: A preliminary examination of its psychometric properties. *Journal of Clinical Child Psychology, 30*, 376-384.

267. Greenwald, R. (2000). *Child Report of Post-Traumatic Symptoms (CROPS) and Parent Report of Post-Traumatic Symptoms (PROPS): Manual and measures.* Baltimore, MD: Sidran.

268. Greenwald, R. & Rubin, A. (1999). Brief assessment of children's post-traumatic symptoms: Development and preliminary validation of parent and child scales. *Research on Social Work Practice, 9*, 61-75.

269. Putnam, F.W. (1988). *Child Dissociative Checklist.* (Available from the author at National Institute of Mental Health, Building 15K, 9000 Rockville Pike, Bethesda, MD 20892-2668).

270. Bryant, R. (2004). Assessing acute stress disorder. In J.P. Wilson & T.M. Keane (Eds.), *Assessing psychological trauma and PTSD, Second Edition,* (pp 45-62). New York: Guilford Publications.

271. Bryant, R.A., Harvey, A.G., Dang, S., & Sackville, T. (1998). Assessing acute stress disorder: Psychometric properties of a structured clinical interview. *Psychological Assessment, 10*, 215-220.

272. Bryant, R.A., Moulds, M., & Guthrie, R. (2000). Acute stress disorder scale: A self-report measure of acute stress disorder. *Psychological Assessment, 12*, 61-68.

273. Cardena, E., Koopman, C., Classen, C., Waelde, L.C., & Spiegel, D., (2000). Psychometric properties of the Stanford Acute Stress Reaction Questionnaire: A valid and reliable measure of acute stress. *Journal of Traumatic Stress, 13*, 719-734.

Index

We Want Your Opinion!

Comments about **Post-Traumatic and Acute Stress Disorders**:

Other titles you would like Compact Clinicals to offer:

To be placed on our mailing list, please provide the following:

Name: _____

Address: _____

E-mail: _____

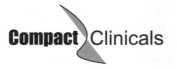

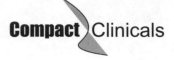

Order in 3 easy steps:

▶ 1   Provide complete billing and shipping information

Name _____   Company _____

Profession _____   Dept./Mail Stop _____

Street Address/P.O. Box _____

City/State/Zip _____

Telephone _____   ☐ Ship to Residence   ☐ Ship to Business

▶ 2   Choose Titles

For Clinicians:	Qty.	Unit Price	Total
Attention Deficit Hyperactivity Disorder *The latest assessment and treatment strategies*		$16.95	
Bipolar Disorder *The latest assessment and treatment strategies*		$16.95	
Borderline Personality Disorder *The latest assessment and treatment strategies*		$16.95	
Conduct Disorders *The latest assessment and treatment strategies*		$16.95	
Depression in Adults *The latest assessment and treatment strategies*		$16.95	
Obsessive Compulsive Disorder *The latest assessment and treatment strategies*		$16.95	
Post-Traumatic and Acute Stress Disorders *The latest assessment and treatment strategies*		$16.95	

For Physicians:

Bipolar Disorder: Treatment and Management		$18.95	

	Subtotal
Continuing Education credits *available for mental health professionals.* *Call 1-800-408-8830 for details.*	**Tax** (In MO ONLY, add 7.975%)
	Shipping ($3.75 first book/ $1.00 per additional book)
	TOTAL

▶ 3   Choose Payment Method

Please charge my: ☐ Visa   ☐ MasterCard   ☐ Discover   ☐ American Express   ☐ Check Enclosed

Account # __ __ __ __ — __ __ __ __ — __ __ __ __ — __ __ __ __   Exp. Date __ __ / __ __

Name on Card _____   Cardholder Signature _____

Postal Orders: Compact Clinicals, 7205 NW Waukomis Dr., Suite A, Kansas City, MO 64151

Telephone Orders: Toll Free 1-800-408-8830   **Fax Orders:** 1(816)587-7198

We Want Your Opinion!

Comments about **Post-Traumatic and Acute Stress Disorders**:

Other titles you would like Compact Clinicals to offer:

To be placed on our mailing list, please provide the following:

Name: _____

Address: _____

E-mail: _____

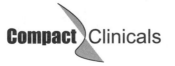

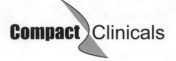

Order in 3 easy steps:

▶ 1 Provide complete billing and shipping information

Name _____ Company _____

Profession _____ Dept./Mail Stop _____

Street Address/P.O. Box _____

City/State/Zip _____

Telephone _____ ☐ Ship to Residence ☐ Ship to Business

▶ 2 Choose Titles

For Clinicians:

	Qty.	Unit Price	Total
Attention Deficit Hyperactivity Disorder *The latest assessment and treatment strategies*		$16.95	
Bipolar Disorder *The latest assessment and treatment strategies*		$16.95	
Borderline Personality Disorder *The latest assessment and treatment strategies*		$16.95	
Conduct Disorders *The latest assessment and treatment strategies*		$16.95	
Depression in Adults *The latest assessment and treatment strategies*		$16.95	
Obsessive Compulsive Disorder *The latest assessment and treatment strategies*		$16.95	
Post-Traumatic and Acute Stress Disorders *The latest assessment and treatment strategies*		$16.95	

For Physicians:

	Qty.	Unit Price	Total
Bipolar Disorder: Treatment and Management		$18.95	

Continuing Education credits available for mental health professionals. Call 1-800-408-8830 for details.

Subtotal	
Tax (In MO ONLY, add 7.975%)	
Shipping ($3.75 first book/ $1.00 per additional book)	
TOTAL	

▶ 3 Choose Payment Method

Please charge my: ☐ Visa ☐ MasterCard ☐ Discover ☐ American Express ☐ Check Enclosed

Account # __ __ __ __ − __ __ __ __ − __ __ __ __ − __ __ __ __ Exp. Date __ __ / __ __

Name on Card _____ Cardholder Signature _____

Postal Orders: Compact Clinicals, 7205 NW Waukomis Dr., Suite A, Kansas City, MO 64151

Telephone Orders: Toll Free 1-800-408-8830   **Fax Orders:** 1(816)587-7198